AF522263

General Veterinary Pathology

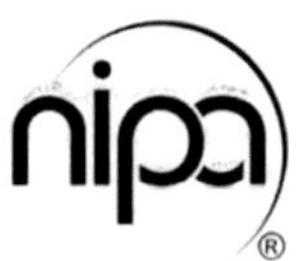

NIPA® GENX ELECTRONIC RESOURCES & SOLUTIONS P. LTD.
New Delhi-110 034

About the Authors

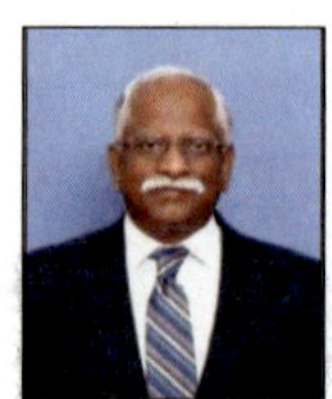

Dr. C. Balachandran was born on 28.07.1957 in Mannargudi town of Tiruvarur District, Tamil Nadu. He obtained B.V.Sc., M.V.Sc. and Ph.D. (Veterinary Pathology) degrees from Madras Veterinary College. He is Charter Member and Diplomat of Indian College of Veterinary Pathologists (ICVP). He is also PG Diploma holder in Agricultural Journalism-PGDAJ and Ethnoveterinary Practices PGDEVP. He started his career at Namakkal in 1980 and promoted as Associate Professor in 1988 and Professor in 1996. He served as Vice- Chancellor of Tamil Nadu Veterinary and Animal Sciences University (TANUVAS) for three years from 09-04-2018. He also served as Registrar of TANUVAS and as the Dean, Madras Veterinary College and Faculty Dean of Veterinary and Animal Sciences, TANUVAS. He has published about 400 scientific articles including 73 articles in International journals. He has worked on skin tumours, mammary tumours, lymphadenopathies, and also pathology of liver, spleen, kidney, stomach, intestine and colon mostly on cytology and histopathology and molecular pathology. He was instrumental in introducing cytological diagnosis of disease in animals. Other areas of research interests are avian diseases, cancer biology , avian mycotoxicosis, toxicopathology and indigenous medicinal effects. He has about 90+ awards to his credit. Notable Awards: University gold medal for the best thesis in avian diseases, Fellow of FAO, FIAVP, FASAW, National Academy of Veterinary Sciences and Tamil Nadu State Scientist Award.

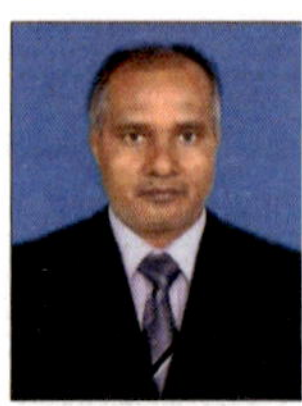

Dr. N. Pazhanivel, M.V.Sc., Ph.D., M.A. (Public Administration), PGDEVP., Diplomate ICVP., FASAW, FIAVP, ICMR DHR IF, and Professor of Pathology, Madras Veterinary College, Chennai-600007. His area of research includes oncology, avian oncogenic viruses, avian pathology, cytopathology, histopathology, fish histopathology and toxicopathology. He has published 322 research articles (International -65; National-257). He has published 64 popular articles. He has presented 323 research papers (International-91; National- 232). He has received 61 awards. He has published 3 books and 56 book chapters. He has completed 6 projects and currently 7 projects are handling. He has completed Post-Doctoral Fellowship Research Training at Pennsylvania State University, USA in 2020. He visited to Liverpool University, United Kingdom for educational training program under ICAR- NAHEP /IDP – TANUVAS during January to February, 2023. He is acting as the Editor, The Indian Veterinary Journal from 2022 onwards. He acted as the Secretary, Indian College of Veterinary Pathologists (ICVP) from 2020 to 2022 and now acting as Registrar, Indian College of Veterinary Pathologists (ICVP) from 2023 onwards.

General Veterinary Pathology

C. Balachandran
N. Pazhanivel

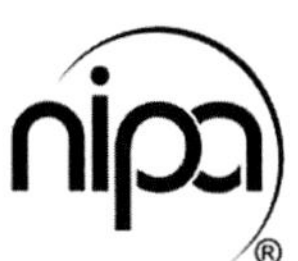

NIPA® GENX ELECTRONIC RESOURCES & SOLUTIONS P. LTD.
New Delhi-110 034

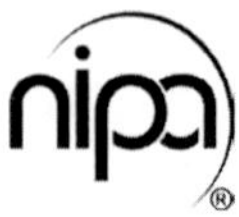

NIPA® GENX ELECTRONIC RESOURCES & SOLUTIONS P. LTD.

101,103, Vikas Surya Plaza, CU Block
L.S.C. Market, Pitam Pura, New Delhi-110 034
Ph : +91-11-43860225, Mob.: +91 9717133558, 9540816132
E-mail: newindiapublishingagency@gmail.com
Website: www.nipaersources.com

Print ISBN: 978-93-58872-91-0

ebook ISBN: 978-93-58873-02-3

NIPA® also publishes books in a variety of electronic formats. Some content that appears in print may not be available in electronic books, and vice versa.

Composed and Designed by NIPA®.

Preface

Pathology is a bridging subject between basic anatomy, physiology and biochemistry and clinical subjects of medicine, surgery and obstetrics and gynecology. Pathology provides understanding of the disease processes underlying each disease condition that is applied in diagnosis, prognosis and treatment of diseases.

Veterinary Pathology is the subject of terminology. One should learn it and have knowledge of it to understand the subject and in future applications and the terms are later phases of learning.

The study of Veterinary Pathology begins with general conditions common to disease processes-systemic and/or special/specific diseases. It is the beginning of learning process in Veterinary Pathology.

General Veterinary Pathology deals about the fundamental processes of diseases of animals that are common to more than one tissue or organ. Study of diseases is an essential component of pathology. Subject in bulleted points and schematic flow diagram.

This book deals about the introduction and scope, causes, haemodynamic derangements, degeneration, necrosis, gangrene, cell injury, pigmentation, calcification, photosensitization, growth disturbances, inflammation, healing and immunopathology.

This book can serve as a quick ready reckoner. This book covers the syllabus as per the VCI Undergraduate Curriculum. It will be useful to students of both under graduate and post graduate level as well as researchers, scientists and Veterinarians.

We are thankful to Tamil Nadu Veterinary and Animal Sciences University (TANUVAS), Chennai for the facilities provided and support.

C. Balachandran
N. Pazhanivel

Contents

1

Introduction and Scope of Veterinary Pathology

Introduction and Scope of Veterinary Pathology

- The aim of study of veterinary and animal sciences is to produce a competent veterinarians. The veterinarians are involved in the diagnosis of diseases of livestock, poultry, wild animals and captive animal species. The study of diseases is essential component of pathology.
- Pathology (Gr. Path(o) - Disease; logos: science, treatise, sum of knowledge in a particular subject)
- Pathology is the subject linking basic subjects of anatomy, histology, embryology, physiology and biochemistry to clinical subjects of medicine, surgery and obstetrics and gynaecology.
- Pathology is a subject of terminology.
- It is important to familiarize with different terminologies used in describing events/ disease conditions. The definition of each terminology is the gateway to understanding the particular disease process.

Definitions-Many

- Pathology literally means study of disease or discourse of disease.
- Pathology is that branch of medicine treating of the essential nature of disease especially of the changes in body tissues and organs which cause or caused by disease (Dorland).
- Pathology is study of the molecular, biochemical, functional and morphological aspects of diseases in the fluids, cells, tissues and organs of the body.
- Summary: Pathology is study of the functional and morphological alterations in tissues and fluids of the body during the disease (Thomson, 1984)

Aetiology

- The science dealing with causes of disease.
- Study of causation of disease

Incubation period

Incubation period is the time period between the action of a cause and manifestation of disease.

Pathogenesis

- Pathogenesis is development of morbid conditions or of disease or mechanism by which the causes produce diseases. e.g. In traumatic reticuloperitonitis/pericarditis in cattle sharp objects like nails ingested are usually trapped in the reticulum.
- Movement of reticulum and pressure from pregnant uterus in cows favours the piercing of foreign body through the wall of the reticulum, setting up reticulitis and then into peritoneal cavity causing injury causing peritonitis and may pierce through diaphragm and apex of the heart setting traumatic pericarditis.
- If the foreign body is carrying pyogenic organisms, it may end in purulent inflammation.

Clinical signs

- Clinical signs are outward manifestations of the patient's suffering from diseases while alive during life.

Lesions

- Lesions are macroscopical (visible to naked eye) or microscopical changes in tissue structure.

Pathognomonic lesion(s)

- Pathognomonic lesion(s) is/are characteristic for a particular disease, seen grossly and or microscopically e.g. Blue tongue in sheep- Haemorrhages in the base of the pulmonary artery and base of the aorta, Johne's disease in cattle- Corrugation of intestine, pasteurellosis in sheep;- disseminated intravascular coagulation (DIC) in lungs

Course of the disease

- Course of the disease is the duration of time through which the series of changes characteristic of disease pass through to their ultimate end.

Termination of disease

- A disease may terminate in recovery or death or may prolong or continue to become a chronic disease.

Diagnosis

- Diagnosis is the art of determination of the nature of disease, its causes, symptoms, lesions etc.

Morphological diagnosis

- Where diagnosis is based on the alterations observed in a tissue or organ. i.e. naming the lesion e.g. Pneumonia (Inflammation of lungs), enteritis (Inflammation of intestine).
- This provides information to clinician on the extent, duration, distribution and type of lesion.

Aetiological diagnosis

- Where specific cause of the disease can be identified i.e. naming the cause. e.g. Cause of pneumonia-Bacteria, virus, fungus, foreign body, Pasteurellosis-*Pasteurella multocida*

Specific or definitive diagnosis

Where the pathognomonic lesions are characteristic of the disease can be observed. i.e. naming the specific entity/disease involved e.g. Corrugated appearance of intestine in Johne's disease in cattle, haemorrhages in the base of the aorta and pulmonary artery in blue tongue in sheep

Differential diagnosis

Differential diagnosis is aimed at diagnosing a disease by differentiating from different diseases based on clinical and pathological findings. This is the first step in diagnosis.

Prognosis

- Prognosis is pronouncing probable/expected outcome of the disease
- Prognosis of a disease is the estimate by a clinician of probable severity and outcome of the disease.

Sequelae

Final end result of the disease

What is autopsy, necropsy and biopsy

Autopsy

- Autopsy is seeing with one's own eyes (Used in human or interchangeably used in Human and Veterinary Medicine).
- The pathologist cuts open a carcass to see the lesions in diseases.

Necropsy

- Necropsy is seeing a corpse (Used in Veterinary Medicine)

Biopsy

- Biopsy is the collection of materials for living animals to diagnosis of diseases.
- Examination of samples collected /obtained from living animals.

What is scope of pathology

- Pathology is aiding in the diagnosis of diseascs.
- Pathology in understanding the disease process.
- Pathology provides base for prognosis, control and rationale treatment and prevention of diseases.

Now let us see the Branches of Pathology

- **General pathology** deals with fundamental diseases processes that are common to more than one tissue or organ
- **Systemic pathology** is study of diseases peculiar to certain systems or organs.
- **Special pathology** is study of diseases caused by specific microbial Pathogens.
- **Clinical pathology** is the branch of pathology used in the diagnosis of the diseases in the hospital at the patient's bedside (Bedside diagnosis).
- **Comparative pathology** is the study of diseases of animals and comparing them to those occurring in humans.

- **Nutritional pathology** is the study of disease processes resulting from deficiency or excess of essential foods.
- **Experimental pathology** means the study of disease artificially produced in animals.
- **Chemical pathology** deals with alterations in biochemical processes in diseases.
- **Oncology** (Gk. Onco-Tumour) is study of tumours.
- **Foreign Animal Diseases (FAD)**: Diseases not occurring in a country but reported in elsewhere in other countries. Scientist study about the diseases by inducing in susceptible species in an isolated environment to understand the disease process for diagnosis and prevention
- **A foreign animal disease (FAD)** is an animal disease or pest, whether terrestrial or aquatic, that is not known to exist in the United States or its territories. When these diseases can have a significant impact on human health or livestock production and when control and eradication efforts would result in significant economic loss, they are considered a threat to the United States. E.g. African swine fever, classical swine fever, contagious bovine pleuropneumonia, Contagious equine metritis, Dourine, Foot-and-mouth disease, Glanders, Rinderpest, Teschen disease and Screwworms (Source: Wikipedia, Internet)
- These are achieved through examination of tissues from living animals (Biopsy) and dead animals/carcass /necropsy or by experimentation.
- Pathology deals with disease processes involving aetiology, pathogenesis and clinical effects of diseases in animals and tries to explain what went wrong.

2

Major Intrinsic and Extrinsic Causes of Disease

Definition

- Aetiology is defined as study of causation of disease.

Classification of Causes

- There are several agents or factors that can produce diseases in animals and can originate from within the body (intrinsic) or outside the body. (extrinsic).

Causes are classified into two categories

1. Predisposing causes (Intrinsic/Endogenous factors)
2. Definitive causes (Extrinsic/Exogenous factors)

Predisposing Causes

- Make the animal susceptible to definitive causes.

These include

- **Heredity**-Inherited- Glycogen storage diseases e.g. Pompe's disease (Lysosomal acid maltase deficiency) in cattle, dog
- **Species**- Rinderpest is found in cattle not in other animals.
- **Breed**-Certain breeds are more susceptible to some diseases than others. Heavier breeds of dogs suffer from bone diseases
- **Age**-Young animals are comparatively more prone for disease than adults, nutritional diseases etc.
- **Sex**-Look for diseases of reproductive organs in respective sex.
- **Colour** (Pigmentation)-Sunburns in melanin deficiency, eye cancer in Hereford cattle

Definitive Causes

- These are actual agents that produce diseases.

These are

Physical Causes

- Trauma-Injuries: Mechanical, Accidents
- Excess heat-Burns
- Excess cold-Frost bite, cold shock
- Radiation-UV irradiation, x-radiation

Chemical Causes

- Acids- HCl, H_2SO_4
- Alkalis-NaOH
- Inorganic chemicals- $HgCl_2$ is nephrotoxic
- Organic chemicals-CCl_4 is hepatotoxic

Viable/Biological Causes

- Bacteria-Anthrax bacilli
- Viruses-Foot and mouth disease virus (Aphthovirus)
- Mycoplasma-respiratory disease in chicken
- Rickettsia-Ehrlichiosis
- Fungus-Dermatomycosis (eg. Dogs-Fungal dermatitis); aspergillosis (e.g. Brooder pneumonia in chicks, emu)
- Parasites-Haemonchosis in ruminants, ascaridiasis (Pups, buffalo calves) and ancylostomosis in dogs

Nutritional Causes

- Excess-Hypervitaminosis A, D- Skin and bone disorders
- Deficiency-Hypoproteinaemia, hypovitamonosis (e.g. Xerophthalmia in vitamin A deficiency, star gazing in chicken in vitamin B1 deficiency; curled toe paralysis in vitamin B2 deficiency), Hypocalcaemia (Milk fever in high yielding cows)

Immunological diseases- Hypersensitivities-Anaphylaxis

Toxins- Phytotoxins, Zootoxins (Snake venom), Pesticides (Organochlorines, organophosphorus compounds etc)

Types of physical (Traumatic) injuries

Perforation is a wound caused by a bullet or nail.

Laceration is a wound in which there is tearing of tissues. e.g: Automobile accidents, road accidents, animal drawn on rough surface.

Concussion is a violent shock caused by an injury and is usually applied to injuries of the head. There may or may not be loss of consciousness.

Sprain is an injury of joint in which there may be stretching or rupture of ligaments, muscles or tendons. In this anatomical relationship of the structures is maintained.

Luxation or dislocation is deviation from its original position in which the anatomical relationship are not maintained and the ligaments may be torn.

Fracture is discontinuity of a bone.

Miscellaneous causes

Iatrogenic disease is a condition produced by the physician by over or needless medication.

Idiosyncrasy (Idio: Self, personal, own; Syncrasy: Happening) is different reaction of animals to drugs. Untoward reaction to drugs

Disturbances in Development (Anomalies & Monster)

- **Anomaly** is a developmental defect affecting an organ or part of the body or
- **Anomaly** is the disturbance of development that involves an organ or a portion of an organ.
- **Monster** is an animal in which extensive abnormal developments are present.
- A **congenital disease** is one in which the patient is born with the disease whereas an inherited disease is one which is due to factors in the genetic materials received from the parents

Classification of Anomalies

A. Arrest of Development

Agenesia is an incomplete and imperfect development of an organ or part and aplasia is absence of an organ or part. That occurs in small portion of patients and have no obvious relationship to drugs and duration of therapy. Target: Liver

- **Acrania** is absence of most or all of the bones of the cranium.
- **Amelia** is absence of one or more limbs.
- **Anencephalia** is absence of the brain.
- **Hypocephalia** is incomplete development of the brain.
- **Hemicrania** is absence of half of the head.
- **Exencephalia** is defective skull with brain exposed or extruded. If the protruding brain contains a ventricle which is filled with excessive amount of fluid, the malformation is a hydrencephalocele.
- **Arhinencephalia** is absence or rudimentary development of the olfactory lobe with corresponding lack of development of the external olfactory organs.
- **Agnathia** is absence of the lower jaw.
- **Anophthalmia** is absence of one or both eyes.
- **Abrachia** is absence of the forelimbs.
- **Abrachiocephalia** is absence of forelimbs and head.
- **Adactylia** is absence of digits.

2. Fissures on the Median line of the Head, Thorax, and Abdomen

- **Cranioschisis** (Fissures in skull)
- **Cheiloschisis** (lip), often referred to as harelip.
- **Palatoschisis** (oral) cavity, often called cleft palate. Harelip and cleft palate result from faulty development of the maxillary process derived from the first visceral arch.
- **Rachischisis** (spinal column fissure).
- **Schistorrachis** or spina bifida (spinal column fissure)
- **Schistothorax** (thorax or sternum fissure).

- **Schistosomus-** A abdomen tissue.
- **Schistocormus** (Thorax, neck or abdominal wall). Results from arrested development of the amnion.

3. Fusion of paired organs

- **Cyclopia** is fused eyes
- **Ren arcuatus** is fused kidneys, often referred to as horse-shoe kidney.
- **Palatoschisis** is fissure of palate

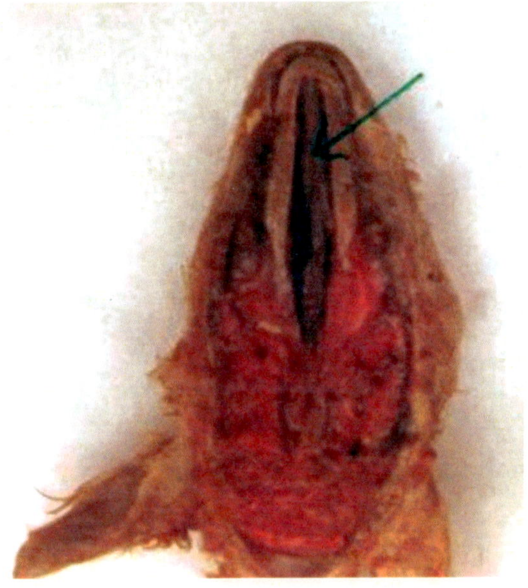

B. Excess of Development Multiple organs

1. **Congenital hypertrophy**: Hemi hypertrophy (partial)
2. Increase in the number of a part

Polyotia (ears), **Polyodontia** (teeth), **Polymelia** (limbs), **Polydactylia** (digits)

Polymastia (mammary gland)

Polythelia (teats)

Displacements During Development

A. Displacements of organs

- **Dextrocardia** is transposition of the heart to the right side.
- **Ectopia cordis** cervicalis is displacement of the heart into the neck.

B. Displacements of tissues

- **Teratoma** is inclusion of multiple displaced and also neoplastic tissue within an individual.
- **Dermoid** is inclusion within an individual of a mass containing skin, hair, feathers, or teeth depending on the species and often arranged as an epidermal cyst (Dermoid cyst).
- **Odontoid cyst** is inclusion within an individual of a mass of dental enamel and cement.
- **Dentigerous cyst** is inclusion within an individual of one or more imperfectly formed teeth.
- **Fusion of sexual characters**
- **Hermaphrodite** is an individual having both testicular and ovarian tissue. Pseudohermaphrodite is an animal having unisexual development of the sex glands (either testicular or ovarian tissue), but having also either a unisexual or bisexual development of the other parts of the genitalia.
- **Freemartin** is a female calf having arrested development of the sex organs and being the twin of perfect male.

Monsters

- A **monster or monstrosity** is a disturbance of development that involves several organs and causes great distortion of the individual.
- For the most part monsters possess a duplication of all or most of the organs and other parts of the body.
- They develop from a single ovum.
- They are therefore the product of incomplete twinning.

Classification of the Monsters

Twins Entirely Separate

- Although separate, these twins are in a single chorion. One twin as a rule is well developed;
- the other is malformed (**acardius**). In the malformed foetus, there is arrested development of the heart, lungs, and trunk.
- Such monsters may lack a head (**acephalus**), limbs and other recognizable features (**amorphous**), or the trunk (**acormus**).

Twins United

- These twins are more or less completely united and are of symmetrical development.

A. Anterior Twinning: The anterior part of the individual is double, the posterior single.

- **Pygopagus** – united in the pelvic region with the bodies side by side.
- **Ischiopagus** – united in the pelvic region with the bodies at an obtuse (not pointed) angle.
- **Dicephalus** – two separate heads; doubling may also affect the neck, thorax and trunk.
- **Diproosopus** – doubling in the cephalic region without complete separation of heads; only the face doubled.

B. Posterior Twinning: The posterior part is double, the anterior single.

- **Craniopagus** – brains usually separated; bodies as a rule at an acute angle.
- **Cephalothoracopagus** – union of head and thorax.
- **Dipygus** – doubling of posterior extremities and posterior part of body.

C. Twinning Almost Complete: Duplication of the whole trunk or the anterior or posterior extremities with parallel, ventral arrangement of the foetuses. The pair is joined in the region of the thorax, and also often in the abdominal region.

- **Thoracopagus** – united only by the thorax.
- **Prosopothoracopagus** – besides the union the thorax the abdomen, the head and neck are united.
- **Rachipagus** – thorax and lumbar portion of the spinal column united.

3

Haemodynamic Disorders

Hyperaemia and Congestion

Definition

Hyperaemia is increased volume of blood in affected tissue or part.

Hyperaemia (Active Hyperaemia)

Occurs in arterioles or arteries

Increased blood flow in capillaries

Congestion (Passive Hyperaemia)

Occurs due to impaired venous drainage

Stasis of blood in veins

classification of hyperaemia

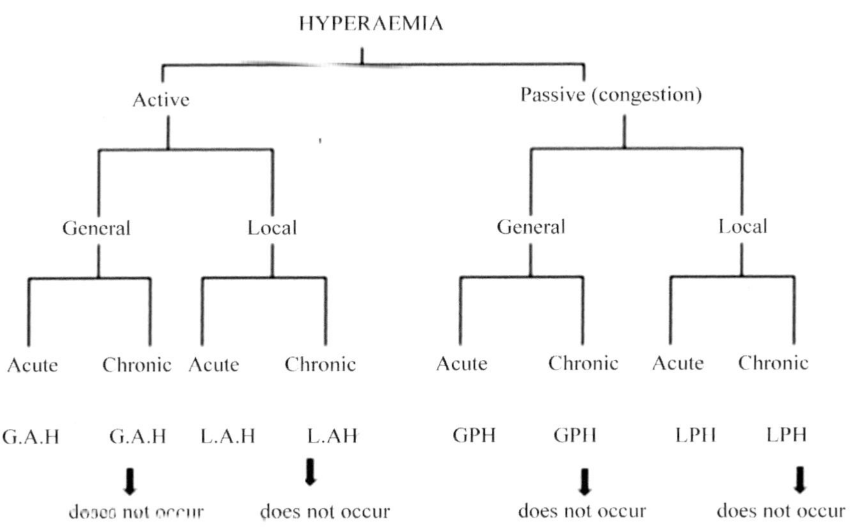

Active Hyperaemia

- Increased blood in arterial side
- Usually due to inflammation
- All active hyperaemia are acute
- Chronic active hyperaemia does not occur
- Occurs when there is a demand for oxygen and nutrients - increase metabolism
- It is beneficial.

Acute General Active Hyperaemia

- Increased blood throughout the body

Causes

- Various systemic diseases

  e.g. Pasteurellosis, swine erysipelas

  -rapidly beating heart → increased blood supply
- Renal diseases - due to retention of fluids

Macroscopically

Bright red color or organs

Microscopically

Arteries and capillaries are dilated with blood

Result

Disappears if cause is removed

Acute Local Active Hyperaemia

- Increased amount of blood in arterial system within a local area (leg, stomach, lung)
- Most common type of hyperaemia

Causes

- Physiological
- Occurs in stomach and intestine following a meal/feeding

- Lactating mammary gland
- Muscles during exercise
- Genital tract during oestrus

Blushing

- Acute inflammation

Macroscopically

- Enlarged, swollen, heavy

↑ Warmth in skin

Microscopically

- In live animals, arteries, arterioles and capillaries are distended with blood
- Difficult to detect in dead animals

Passive Hyperaemia (or Congestion)

Increased blood in the venous end due to improper drainage.

Grneral

- if interference is central (i.e.) lungs, heart

Local

- Involve vein of an organ or body
- It can be acute or chronic

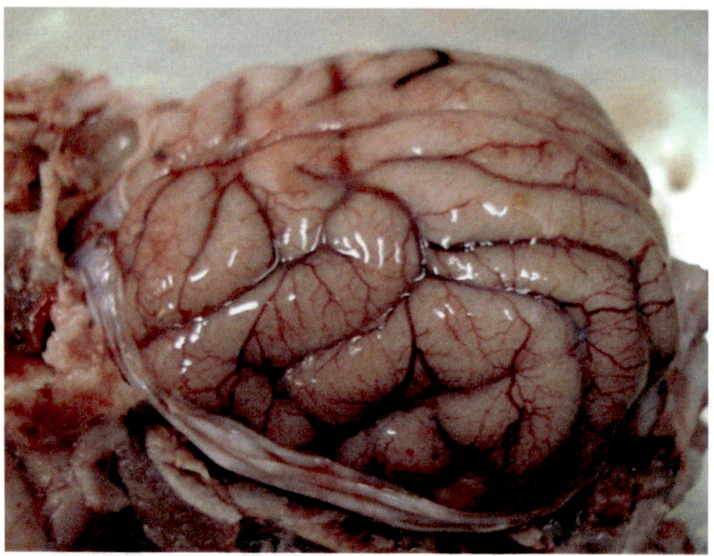

Brain congestion

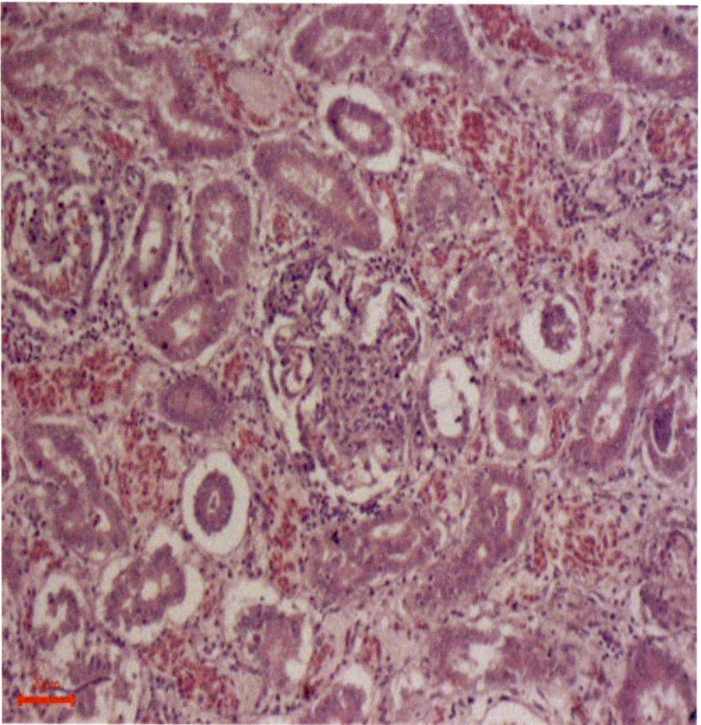

Kidney-Congestion-Chicken

Chronic Venous Congestion (CVC) is More Common

Acute General Passive Hyperaemia

Increase in the amount of blood on the venous side of circulatory system. Occurs due to sudden obstruction to the flow of blood in heart and lungs.

Causes

1. **Heart Failure**

   Degeneration and necrosis of myocardium

   Myocardial infarction

2. **Pneumonia**
3. **Pulmonary Thrombosis or Embolism**
4. **Hydropericardium, Haemopericardium etc**
5. **Hydrothorax, Haemothorax etc**

Macroscopically

- Organs are blue in color (presence of unoxygenated blood)
- Veins distended with blood
- Organs enlarged, heavy
- Upon incision, blood oozes out

Result

- If causes are mild recovery occurs
- If causes are severe death occurs

Chronic General Passive Hyperaemia

Increased blood on venous end persisting for long period of time causes permanent changes (fibrosis, atrophy).

Causes Due to Central Lesions in Heart and Lungs

1. Heart Lesions

- Stenosis of valvular openings

2. Valvular Insufficiency

- Failure of cusps of valves to close property
- Inflammatory tissue
- Thrombus

3. Myocardial Failure

Degeneration and necrosis of muscles
Contraction of muscles affected
↓
Blood pushed in arteries
↓
But accumulates in venous side

4. Anomalies of Heart

Persistent foramen ovale
↓
Interventricular septal defects
↓
Blood moves from one chamber to another
↓
Arterial blood pressure maintained
↓
Blood accumulates in venous end.

5. Constrictive Lesions in Pericardium

- Traumatic pericarditis in cattle

6. Lesions of Lungs

- Obliteration of capillary bed in lungs
- Prevents free flow of blood through the lungs
- Retards flow through right side of heart
- Blood back flows into liver

Causes

- Chronic alveolar pulmonary emphysema in horses (BROKEN WIND)
- Pneumonia
- Hydrothorax, haemothorax
- Compression of major pulmonary vessels
- Tumours

Chronic Venous Congestion is "More Common"

Acute Local Passive Hyperamia

Increase in blood in the veins of a portion (foot, tail, kidney etc) due to sudden obstruction to blood flow

Causes

- Malposition of viscera

  Volvulus, intussusception, torsion

- External pressure

  Ligatures, tourniquets, bandages, abscesses, cysts, haematoma

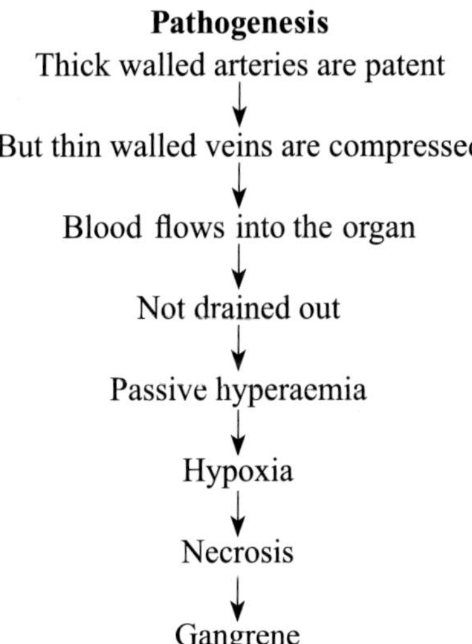

Hypostatic Congestion

Accumulation of blood in ventral portions of the body due to gravity.

Causes

- Occurs in heart diseases
- Recumbency
- Inactive animals
- Large animals
- Heart failure - Agonal Congestion

Appearances

- Veins in ventral portion or organs distended with blood
- Lungs - increase capillary bed
- Intestine and kidneys – necrosis and gangrene
- Causes pneumonia and gangrene of intestine

Significance

- Indicates the side of animals which was ventral at the time of death
- Heart was not able to pump properly
- Location of body in medico–legal cases

Pathology

Veins are engorged with blood
↓
Necrosis of endothelial cells
↓
Haemorrhage

Chronic Local Passive Hyperaemia

Increase in amount of blood for a long time in veins

Permanent tissue changes (atrophy, fibrosis)

Causes

External pressure

- Tumors, abscesses

Obstruction from within

- Thrombus (blood clot)
- Enlarged initially later undergoes atrophy
- Veins - bluish blood
- Oedema due to increase permeability of capillaries
- Fibrosis

Haemorrhage

Definition

Haemorrhage is the escape of blood from a vessel.

Two types

1. Haemorrhage may occur by **rhexis**: When there is rupture of a blood vessel
2. Haemorrhage by **diapedesis** : When blood leaves (RBCs) through intact blood vessels

Site of Haemorrhage

Nomenclature

- **Epistaxis**-Bleeding from nose
- **Haematemesis**-Blood in vomit
- **Haemoptysis**-Blood in sputum
- **Enterorrhagia**-Bleeding from intestine
- **Melena**-Blood in stools
- **Haematuria**-Blood in urine
- **Haemothorax**-Blood in thoracic cavity
- **Haematocoel**-Bleeding into tunica vaginalis
- **Hemosalphinx**-Bleeding in oviducts
- **Metrorrhagia**-Bleeding from uterus
- **Hematoma**-Tumour-like accumulation of blood
- **Apoplexy**-Haemorrhage into brain

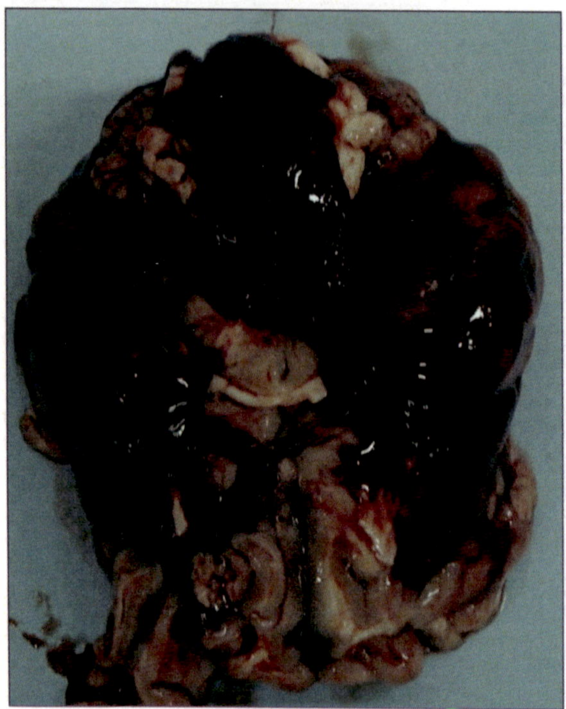

Apoplexy – Bleeding in brain

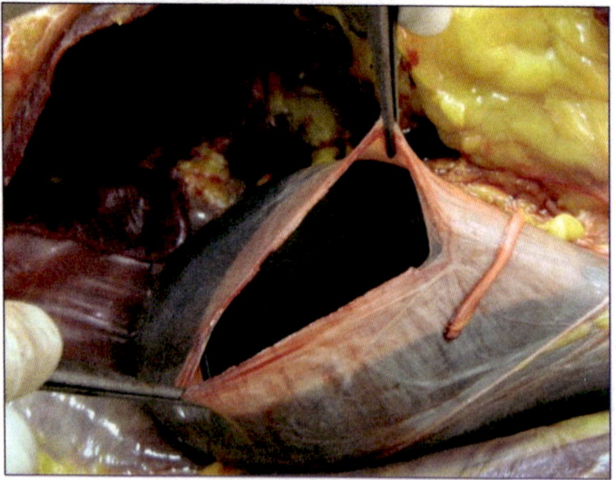

Haemoglobinuria-Coffee, coke, brown coloured urine in urinary bladder-Canine leptospirosis

Size of Haemorrhage

Petechiae: minute; pinpoint haemorrhage

Purpura: approximately 1cm in size bleeding

Ecchymoses: 1 – 2 cm in size bleeding

Extravasation: Larger area of bleeding

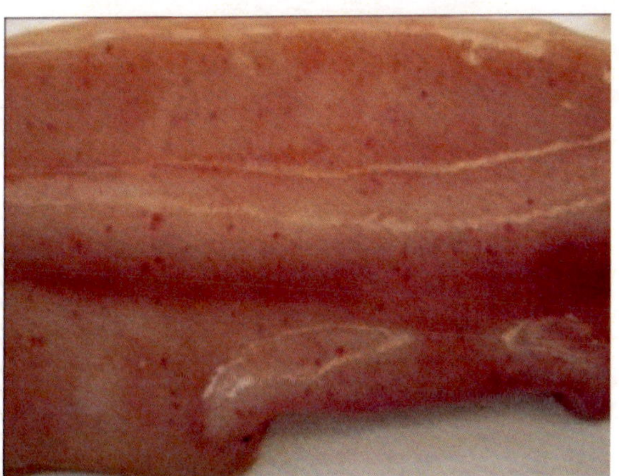

Petechiae -Intestine

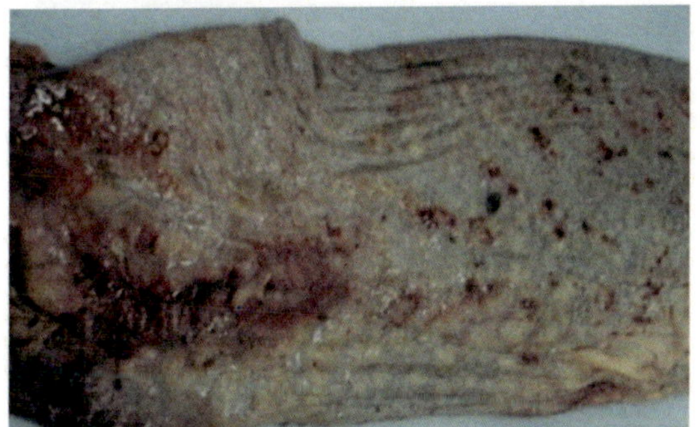

Purpura -Spleen

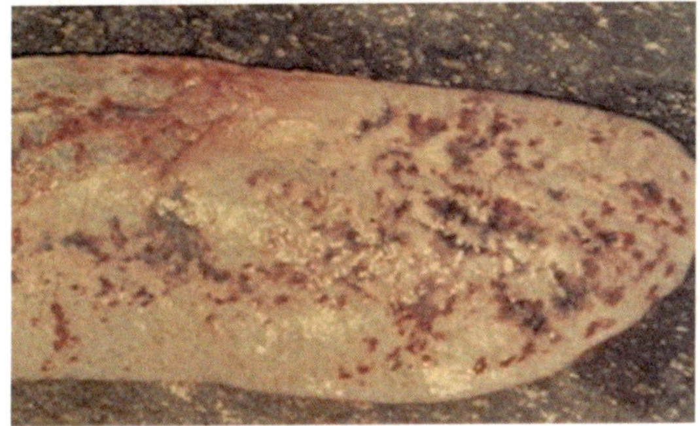

Ecchymoses - Spleen

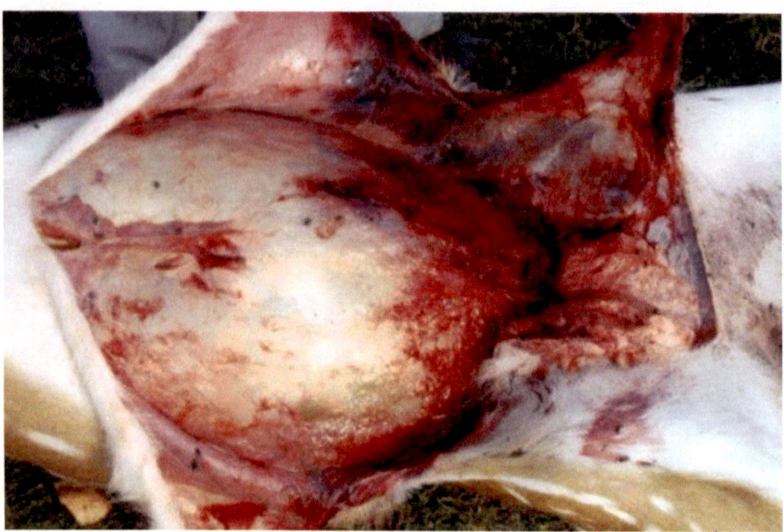

Extravasation- Abdominal viscera

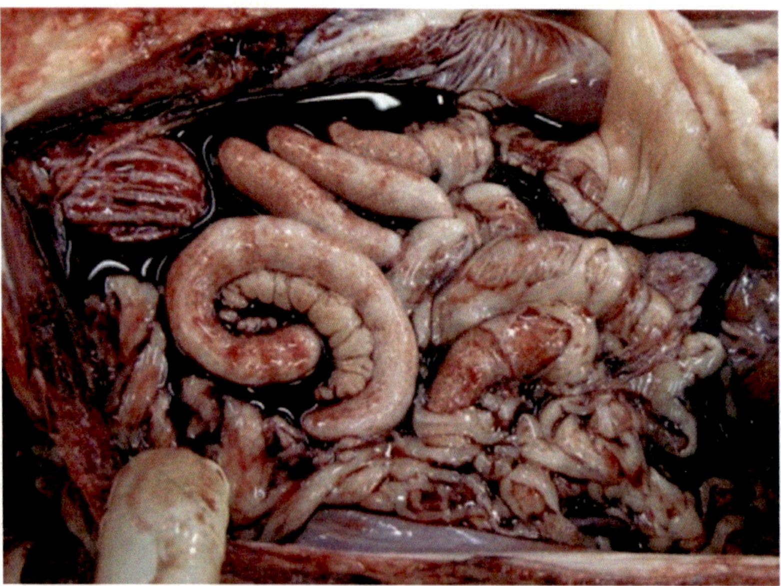

Internal haemorrhage - Abdominal cavity

Source of Haemorrhage

- Cardiac
- Arterial

- Venous
- Capillary

Causes

- Conditions affecting the blood vessels
- Conditions affecting the blood

Conditions of affecting Blood Vessels

- Trauma : Lacerations, incisions, contusions
- Clumps of bacteria, swine erysipelas, anthrax, haemorrhagic septicaemia
- Necrosis of vessel wall
- Ulcers in gastric mucosa
- Neoplasms

Diseases of Vessel Walls

- Aneurysm

  e.g. *Strongylus vulgaris* infection in horses
- Athcroma
- Toxic injury to capillary endothelium
- Bacterial : Anthrax, haemorrhagic septicaemia, black quarter
- Viral : Hog cholera
- Chemicals : Arsenic, phosphorus, chloroform, cyanide
- Enterotoxins : Sheep & calves – *Clostridium welchii* - Asphyxia
- Increased blood pressure
- Excessive exercise → increased blood pressure → Rupture of blood vessel
- Vessel seen in race horses

- **Hypoxia and Lack of Nutrition**
  - Passive venous congestion → damage to endothelium

    ↓

    Haemorrhage

Conditions Affecting Blood Constituents

Haemophilia: Hereditary sex linked disease; Delayed dotting Thrombocytopenic Purpura : Decrease in platelets seen in toxaemias

Nutrition

- Deficiency of vitamin K

- Decreased vitamin K ⟶ decreased prothrombin ⟶ No clotting

Increased use of sulpha drugs ⟶ decreased intestinal microflara

↓

Decreased vitamin K synthesis

Deficiency of vitamin C

Defective formation of ground substance

↓

Capillary endothelium - fragile

↓

Haemorrhage

Heparin Old State
Anaphylactic Shock
and Irradiation increase in heparin * impairs clotting

Plant Toxins

Bracken fern; sweet clover - prevent prothrombin formation

↓

No clotting

Microscopical Appearance

- Presence of erythrocytes outside blood vessels
- Recent haemorrhage stains deeply
- Haemorrhage disintegrates due to action of tissue enzymes

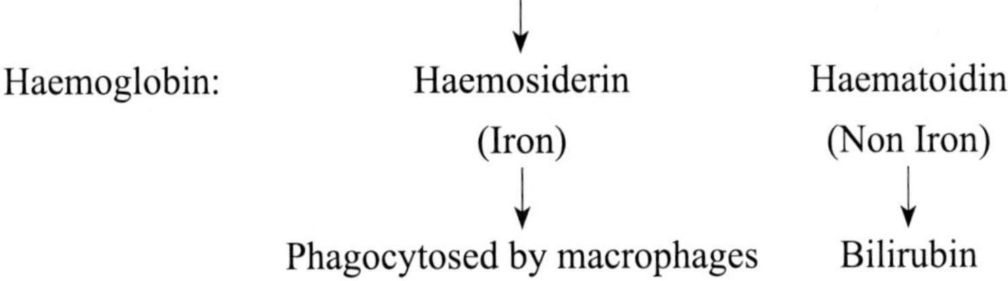

Prussian blue Reaction to Demonstrate Iron

Significance and Result

a. Depends on volume, rate. site.

Sudden loss of about 30% of blood volume

or

Slow losses of large volume of blood

↓

No clinical significance

(e.g.) Stomach worm infection

b. Site of haemorrhage is very important. Small haemorrhage in brain is **FATAL** whereas small haemorrhage in skeletal muscle or subcutaneous tissue is **Not Fatal**.

Haemorrhage in pericardial sac (Cardlac Tamponade) ⟶ Fatal

c. Iron deficiency anaemia- due to repeated and chronic loss of blood from external surface

d. When erythrocytes are retained in body cavities, joints. tissues

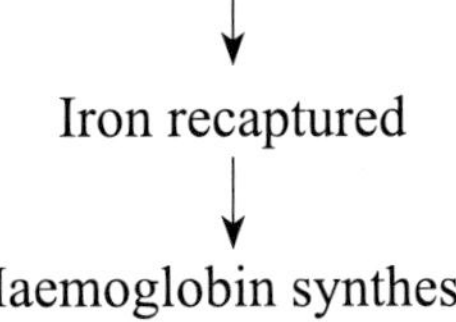

Fate of Haemorrhage

In small haemorrhage, fluid portion is reabsorbed, WBCs move into blood vessels and RBCs phagocytosed. In larger haemorrhage, RBCs are broken down to Hb which is then cleaved to haematoidin and haemosiderin.

Arrest Haemorrhage

Vascular contraction	Small blood vessels
Platelet aggregation	White clot
Clot formation	Red clot → When blood flow is slow
Tissue pressure	Increased perivasular pressure in tissue Decreased intra vascular pressure
Decreased blood pressure	Large harmorrhage Decreased BP No bleeding

Oedema

Definition

Abnormal accumulation of fluid in the intercellular tissue spaces or body cavities

Localized : Due to obstruction of venous outflow – leg

Generalized : Chronic venous congestion or heart failure

Terms used to Describe Oedema

Anasarca: Generalized subcutaneous oedema

Ascites: Fluid in peritoneal cavity

Hydrothorax : Oedematous fluid in thorax

Hydropericardium : Oedematous fluid in pericardium

Oedema is of two types, INFLAMMATORY and NON – INFLAMMATORY oedema

Mechanism of Oedema Formation

Two forces called "**STARLING'S FORCES** "

Filtration Force: Expels fluid from the vessel

Absorption force: Draws fluid into the vessel

We begin with normal fluid balance then to pathology of oedema

Physiology of Fluid Balance

Arterial End

Hydrostatic pressure at arterial end = 45 mm of Hg of capillary (-)

Osmotic pressure of blood due to albumin / globulin = 30mm of Hg

15mm of Hg

Fluid is expelled into the intercellular space (filtration force)

Venous End

Hydrostatic pressure of blood	= 15mm of Hg	(-)
Osmotic pressure of blood	= 30mm of Hg	
Absorption force	15mm of Hg	

Fluid absorbed into capillaries (Absorptive force)

Causes of Oedema

- Decreased plasma osmotic pressure
- Increased hydrostatic pressure
- Increased permeability of vascular endothelium
- Lymphatic obstruction

1. Decreased Plasma Osmotic Pressure- Hypoproteinemia

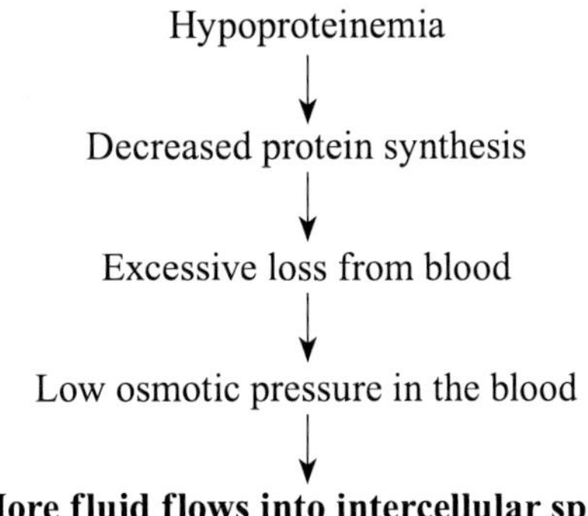

Hydrostatic pressure at arterial end	= 45 mm Hg	(-)
Osmotic pressure at arterial end	= 20 mm Hg	
Rate of fluid flow into tissues	25 mm Hg	
Osmotic pressure at venous end	= 20 mm Hg	(-)
Hydrostatic pressure at venous end	= 15 mm Hg	
Rate of fluid flow into vein	5 mm Hg	

Net Result: 25-5=20 mm Hg rate of fluid accumulates in tissues

Decreased Plasma Osmotic Pressure Mostly Results in Generalised and Severe Oedema

Malnutrition

Advanced Hepatic Disease (Cirrhosis): There is no protein synthesis and so this type of oedema is called **Nutritional or Cachectic Oedema**.

Loss of protein through intestine and stomach in case of stomach worms infection leading to parasitic oedema

In kidney or renal amyloidosis, blood is lost in urine resulting **in Renal Oedema**

Pathogenesis of oedema formation due to Increased Hydrostatic Pressure

2. Increased Hydrostatic Pressure

General or passive hyperaemia ⟶ venous stasis

Central lesion in heart or lungs

or

Local obstruction in a vein

Hydrostatic pressure at arterial end	= 45mm Hg
	(-)
Osmotic pressure at arterial end	= 30mm
Hg Rate of fluid flow into tissues	15mm Hg
Osmotic pressure at venous end	= 30mm Hg
	(-)
Hydrostatic pressure at venous end	= 25mm Hg
Rate of fluid flow in to vein	10mm Hg

Net Result: 5mm Hg rate of fluid accumulates in tissues.

This type of oedema is mild

Mainly the cause is in the heart

Hence Called "**Cardiac Edema**"

3. Increased Permeability of Capillary Endothelium

Due to venous stasis, there is increased hydrostatic pressure

4. Lymphatic Obstruction

Causes

- Tumours, cyst, abscess, bandages, thrombi
- Parasites (*Demodex canis*, mites)
- Filariasis – *Wucheria bancrofti* in humans
- Inflammatory conditions – e.g. farcy; ulcerative lymphangitis in Lymphatic obstruction, fluid and protein accumulates in intercellular space with No drainage resulting in Oedema called **LYMPHOEDEMA**"

Hydrostatic pressure at arterial end = 45 mm Hg Osmotic pressure at arterial end = 25 mm Hg Rate of fluid flow into tissue = 20 mm Hg Osmotic pressure at venous end = 25 mm Hg Hydrostatic pressure at venous end = 15 mm Hg Rate of fluid flow into vein=10 mm Hg

Net Result: 20-10=10 mm Hg rate of fluid accumulates in tissues

5. Sodium Retention

Causes are congestive heart failure, nephrosis/nephritis and acute renal failure. Failure to excrete sodium in urine so water will be retained leading to generalized oedema

Causes of Edema

Increased Vascular Permeability

Vascular leakage associated with inflammation

Infectious agents

- Viruses (e.g., influenza and other respiratory viruses, canine adenovirus 1, equine and porcine Arterivirus, Morbillivirus)
- Bacteria (e.g., Clostridium sp., Shiga-like toxin-producing *Escherichia coli*, *Erysipelothrix rhusiopathiae*)
- Rickettsia (e.g.. *Ehrlichia ruminantium*, *Neorickettsia risticii*. *Anaplasma phagocytophilum*, *Rickettsia rickettsi*)

Immune-mediated

- Type III hypersensitivity (e.g., feline infectious peritonitis, purpura hemorrhagica)

Neovascularization

Anaphylaxis (e.g., type I hypersensitivity to vaccines, venoms, and other allergens)

Toxins (e.g., endotoxin, paraquat, noxious gases, zootoxins)

Clotting abnormalities (e.g., pulmonary embolism, disseminated intravascular coagulation-DIC)

Metabolic abnormalities (e.g., microangiopathy caused by diabetes mellitus, encephalomalacia caused by thiamine deficiency)

Increased Intravascular Hydrostatic Pressure

Portal hypertension (e.g. right-sided heart failure, hepatic fibrosis) Pulmonary hypertension (e.g. left-sided heart failure, high altitude disease) Localized venous obstruction (e.g. gastric dilation and volvulus, intestinal volvulus and torsion, uterine torsion or prolapse. venous thrombosis) Fluid overload (e.g. iatrogenic, sodium retention with renal disease) Hyperaemia (e.g. inflammation, physiologic).

Decreased Intravascular Osmotic Pressure

Decreased albumin production (e.g. malnutrition or starvation, debilitating diseases, severe hepatic disease)

Excessive albumin loss (e.g. gastrointestinal disease [protein losing enteropathies] or parasitism [haemonchosis or trichostrongylosis in sheep], renal disease [protein-losing nephropathies], severe burns)

Water intoxication (e.g., hemodilution caused by sodium retention, salt toxicity)

Decreased Lymphatic Drainage

Lymphatic obstruction or compression (e.g. inflammatory or neoplastic masses, fibrosis)

Congenital lymphatic aplasia or hypoplasia

Intestinal lymphangiectasia

Lymphangitis (e.g., paratuberculosis, sporotrichosis, epizootic lymphangitis of horses)

Pathophysiologic condition of oedema

Increased Hydrostatic Pressure

Impaired venous return

Congestive heart failure

Constrictive pericarditis

Ascites (hepatic cirrhosis)

Venous obstruction or compression

Thrombosis

External pressure (e.g. mass – space occupying diseases)

Lower extremity in activity with prolonged dependency

Arteriolar Dilation

Heat

Neurohumoral dysregulation

Reduced Plasma Osmotic Pressure (Hypoproteinemia) Protein - losing glomerulopathies (nephrotic syndrome) Hepatic cirrhosis (ascites)

Malnutrition

Protein-losing gastroenteropathy

Lymphatic Obstruction

Inflammatory

Neoplastic

Postsurgical

Postirradiation

Sodium Retention

Excessive salt intake with renal insufficiency

Increased tubular reabsorption of sodium

Renal hypoperfusion

Increased renin-angiotensin-aldosterone secretion

Transudate

Transudate contains fluids that pass through a membrane or squeeze through tissue or into the extracellular space of tissues and thin and watery and contain few cells or proteins. Effusion (L. effusio a pouring out) of fluid into extracellular space i.e. Intercellular space, body cavities

Exudate

Exudate contain fluids, cells, or other cellular substances that are slowly discharged from blood vessels usually from inflamed tissues.

Differences Between Transudate and Exudate

S. No.	Characters	Transudate	Exudate
1.	Colour	Clear, water like pale yellow	Cloudy, white, yellow-red
2.	Consistency	Thin, watery no tissue fragments	Thick, creamy, contains tissue fragments
3.	Odour	None	Have odour
4.	pH	Alkaline	Acidic
5.	Specific gravity	1.015 or less	1.018 or higher
6.	Protein	Low, < 3%	High > 4%
7.	Cell count	Low	High, RBCs, WBCs
8.	Enzyme count	Low	High
9.	Bacteria	None	Present
10.	Inflammation	None	Present

Different Types of Oedema

1. Inflammatory oedema
2. Cardiac oedema
3. Renal oedema
4. Hunger / Famine / War oedema
5. Pulmonary oedema
6. Cachetic oedema
7. Myxoedema
8. Parasitic oedema
9. Angioneurotic oedema
10. Brisket disease

1. Inflammatory Oedema

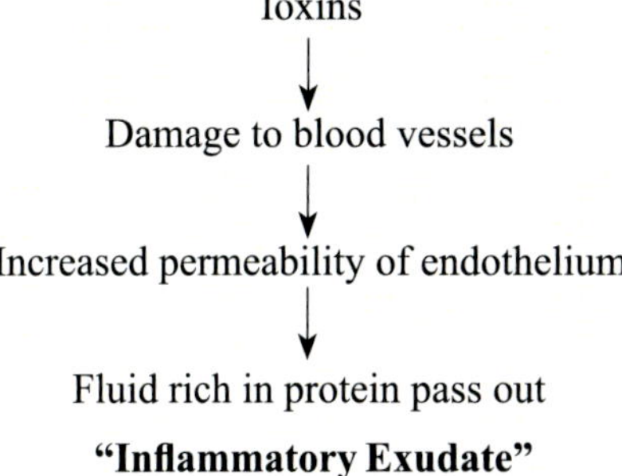

2. Cardiac Oedema

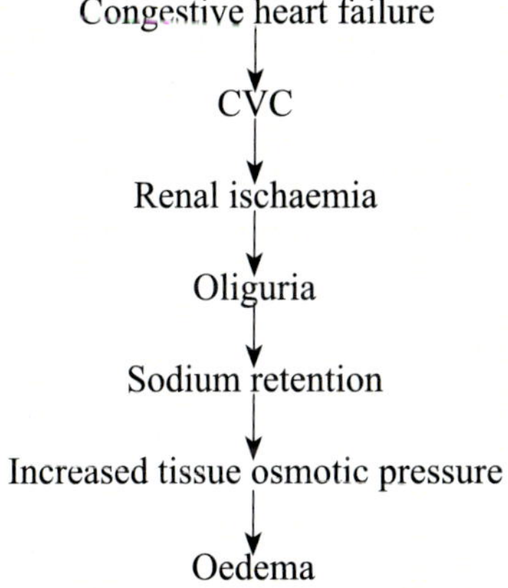

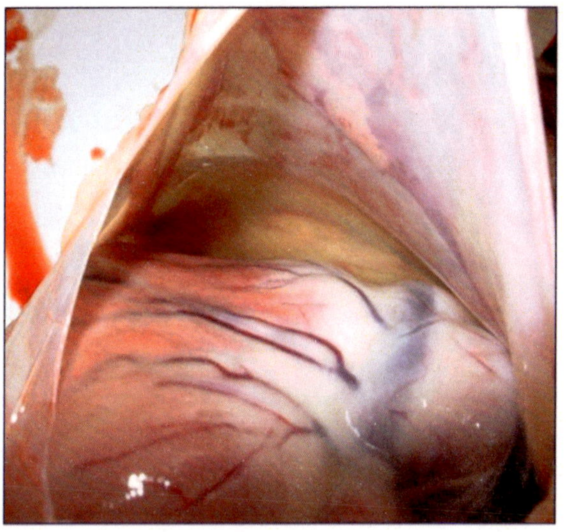

Dog-Oedema-Heart-Hydropericardium- Serous exudate

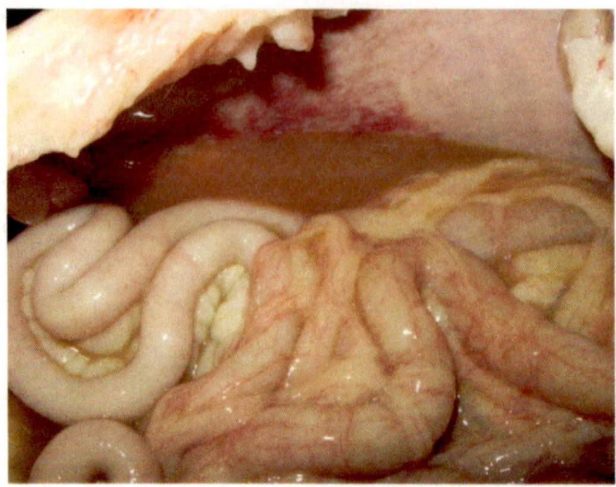

Oedema-Abdominal Cavity -Ascites

Causes for Cardiac Oedema

- Increased hydrostatic pressure of blood
- Increased vascular permeability
- Sodium retention

Symptoms

Oedema of dependent parts

Traumatic pericarditis in bovines

Chronic vesicular emphysema in horses

3. Renal Oedema

Acute glomerulonephritis (in man)

Oedema in face and eyelids

Causes

Decreased plasma osmotic pressure of blood

Toxins
↓
Damage glomerular capillaries
↓
Albuminuria
↓
Hypoproteinaemia

Increased osmotic pressure of ECF

Acute nephritis
↓
Oliguria / Anuria
↓
Sodium retention

Increased capillary permeability

Increased hydrostatic pressure in capillaries in venous side

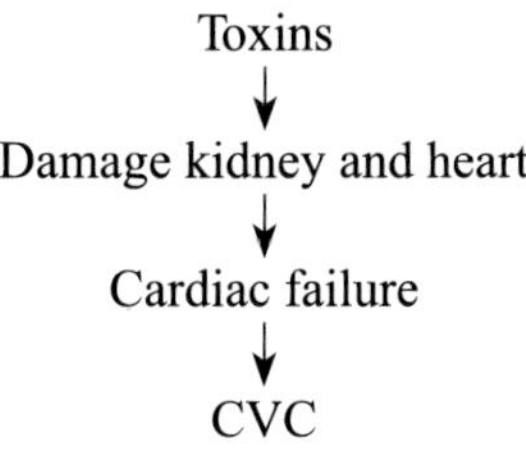

Subacute Nephritis and Nephrosis

Decreased plasma osmotic pressure of blood
↓
Increased sodium retention
↓
Hypoalbuminaemia
↓
Stimulates adrenal cortex
↓
Increased aldosterone increased sodium retention
↓
Chronic glomerulonephritis
↓
Hypertension for long period
↓
Heart failure
↓
CVC
↓
Increased blood pressure in capillaries

4. Hunger / Famine / War Oedema

- War / famine → Decreased protein availability and intake
- Hypoproteinaemia → Decreased plasma osmotic pressure

5. Pulmonary oedema

Causes

- Cardiac failure - hypertension; valvular disease - pericarditis
- Renal lesions
- Pressure on pulmonary veins by neoplasm
- Injury to brain
- Rapid removal of effusion from pleural / peritoneal cavity
- Poisons
- Infections

6. Cachectic Oedema (Protein loss/deficiency)

- Anaemia
- Wasting diseases
- Malnutrition
- Cardiac illness

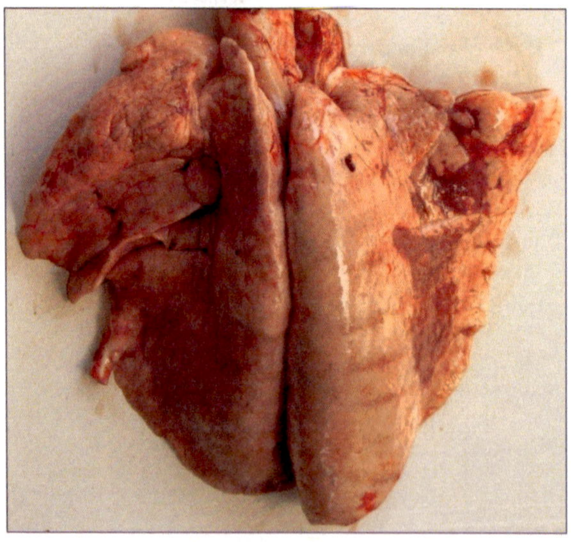

Oedema-Lung-Note: Rib Markings on oedematous lungs

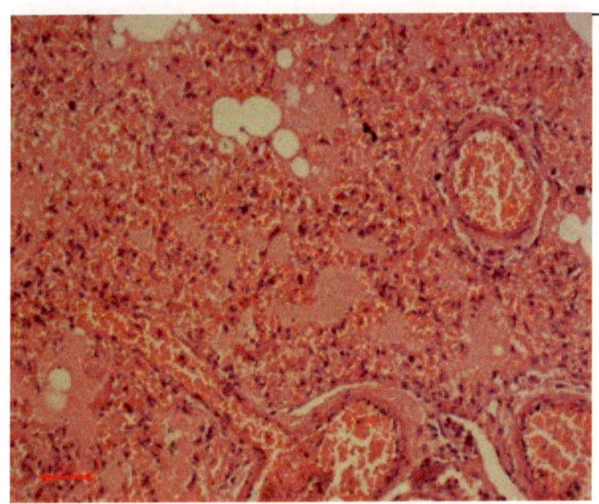

Pulmonary oedema-Dog

7. Myxoedema

Chronic thyroid deficiency
↓
Increased protein accumulation in tissue fluid
↓
Increased osmotic pressure of fluid
↓
Water drawn into site

8. Parasitic Oedema

Stomach worms, liver flukes, amphistomes
↓
Migratory life of cercaria
↓
Haemorrhage & necrosis
↓
Adults in bile duct
↓
Cirrhosis
↓
Decreased protein synthesis
↓
Oedema

Accumulation of fluid in lower jaw "**Bottle Jaw**"

9. Angioneurotic Oedema

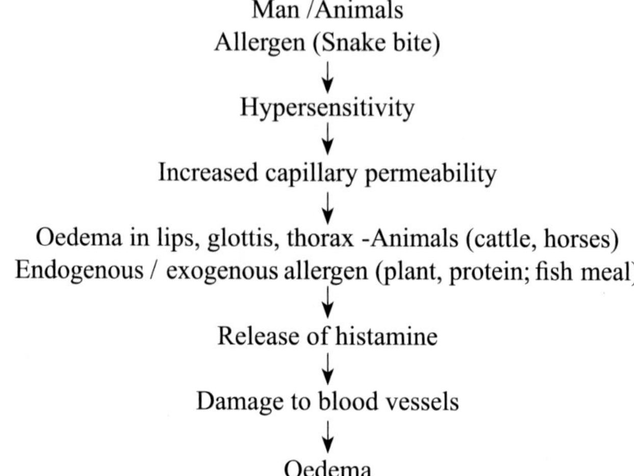

10. Brisket Disease

Cattle moved to high altitude 9000ft above sea level develop oedema in abdomen, brisket, neck, jowl.

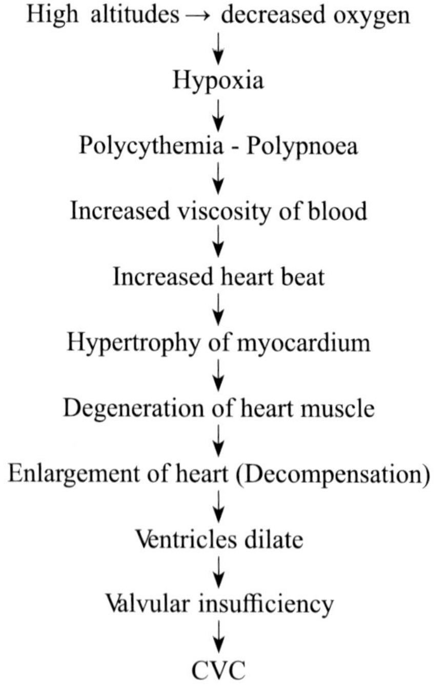

Hypoxia injures capillary endothelium

CVC

Increased BP in capillaries and Hypoxia

hypoxia

Macroscopical Appearance

- Swollen, increase in weight of organs
- Cold due to decrease blood, flow and increase heat dissipation
- Less color
- No pain
- Incision of oedematous organs results in flow of fluid from cut surface
- Pits on pressure
- Fibrosis

Microscopical Appearance

- Space between adjacent cells widened
- During life space filled with fluid
- H&E stain - fine granular material
  - stains faintly pink
  - ↑ pink if ↑ protein
- Atrophy of parenchymatous cells
- Fibrosis - chronic cases

Significance and Result

- Disappears if cause is removed
- Oedema in lung and brain are fatal
- Subcutaneous oedema impairs wound healing

Thrombosis

Formation of clotted mass of blood within the cardiovascular system

Intravascular and intravital clotting of blood

Clotted mass - Thrombus (singular)

- Thrombi (plural)

Differences Between Thrombus and Blood Clot

Thrombus	Blood Clot
Formation Blood vessels Platelets Blood clotting system	Blood clotting system
Composition Platelets Fibrin	Only fibrin
Prognosis Life threatening	Life saving

Causes for Thrombosis

Injury to Endothelium

Trauma : Lacerations, contusions, ruptures, i/v injection Toxins : Streptococci, erysipelothrix (vegetations) Degenerations : Atherosclerosis (damage to intima) Viruses : Hog cholera virus

Parasites : *Strongylus vulgaris* in anterior mesenteric artery in horses

Tumours : Invading tumours

Mechanism of Thrombus Formation

- Active
- Passive

Active Mechanism

Antithrombotic factors and prothrombotic factors are seen on surface of endothelium.

These factors balance between thrombosis and antithrombosis as required.

Anti Thrombotic Factors (present on endothelial cells)

- Inhibit thrombosis

1) Anticoagulant properties

Thrombo modulin and heparin protect against action of thrombin which converts fibrinogen into fibrin

2) Anti platelet properties

- Inhibit platelet aggregation

  Prostacyclin (PGI2)

  Nitric oxide (NO2)

3) Fibrinolytic properties

- Tissue plasminogen activator (tPAs)
- Promotes fibrinolytic activity in blood

Thrombotic Factors

Tissue factor (Thromboplastin)

- Present on endothelium in small amounts
- Activate extrinsic clotting pathway

Stimulated by

- Endotoxins
- Cytokines (IL – 1)
- Tumour necrosis factor (TNF)

von Willebrand factor (vWF)

Protein helps in platelet adherence leading to thrombus formation

Platelet Activating Factor (PAF)- Helps in platelet aggregation leading to thrombus formation

Inhibitor of Plasminogen Activator- Prevents fibrinolysis leading to thrombus formation

Normal Homeostasis: Balance between antithrombotic and prothrombotic factors is maintained in normal endothelium.

Thrombus Formation

Increase in prothrombotic factors and decrease in antithrombotic factors

Passive Mechanism

Endothelium is thromboresistant.

Subendothelial connective tissue is highly thrombogenic.

Subendothelial connective tissue consists of collagen, elastic, fibrinonectin, laminin glycosaminoglycans, thrombosporin

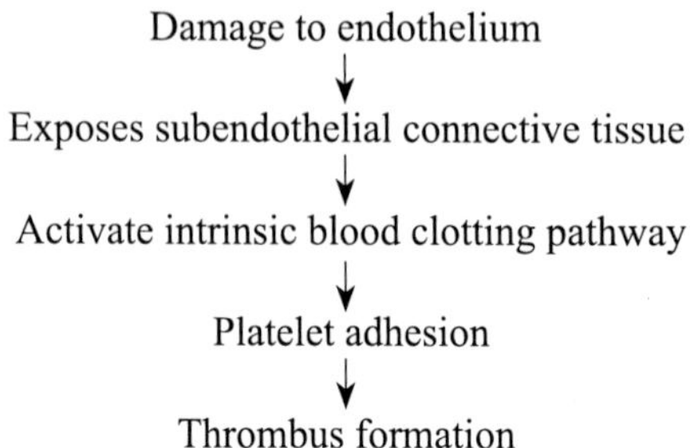

Alterations in Constituents of Blood

Increase in number of platelets

- Parturition
- Surgery

Increase in adhesiveness of platelets

- Parturition
- Surgery

Decrease in heparin (anticoagulant) in diseases

Increased plasma fibrinogen and prothrombin

- Trauma

Increased viscosity of blood

- Dehydration
- Polycythemia

Sludging of blood

- Clumping of cells

Increased fragility of RBCs

Increased cortisone therapy – Rheumatoid arthritis

Increase blood lipids

Increased platelet aggregation

Coronary thrombosis

4. Alterations in Normal Blood Flow

Slowing of blood flow leads to platelet aggregation

Turbulence damages endothelium

- Arterial thrombus
- Venous thrombus
- Cardiac thrombus

5. Causes for Slowing of Blood

- Chronic venous congestion leads to venous stasis
- Old and debilitated animals
- Varicose veins

Common Sites for Thrombosis

Animals

- **Scrotal plexus** - horses
- **Vascular sinuses** – horse and cows (Nasal passage)
- **Large veins of broad ligament of uterus** – cow
- **Anterior mesenteric artery** - horses

Humans

- Leg veins – Congestive heart failure, bed ridden patients

Events in Thrombus Formation-Pathogenesis

Injury to endothelium

↓

Exposes

Highly thrombogenic subendothelial connective tissue

↓

Release of tissue factor-Thromboplastin

↓

Platelet adhesion

↓

Contact activation

(i.e. Shape change, release reaction, further aggregation of platelets)

Adherent & activation of platelets

↓

Platelet reaction occurs in minutes

↓

Enlarge in size

↓

Formation of temporary or primary haemostatic plug

↓

Reversible

Release of tissue factors + Platelet factors

↓

Activates coagulation system

↓

Generate thrombin

(Powerful platelet activator-Agonist

Agonist: A chemical substance capable of combining with a receptor and initiating a reaction)

↓

Platelet contraction

↓

Induced by

Thrombin+ADP for platelets+TxA2 (Prostaglandin) Synthesized by platelets

↓

Mediated by intraplatelet actinomysin with

↓

Fusion of platelets

"**Viscous metamorphosis**"

↓

Leading to **definitive or permanent haemostatic plug**

↓

Irreversible

Thrombin also converts

↓

Fibrinogen to fibrin

(Acting like cement (mortar) to build "Platelet-bricks"

↓

Which further stabilizes plug via fibronectin, attaches to its site of origin

↓

Platelets accumulate at endothelial surface

↓

Form white or buff or pale coloured mass

↓

White or pale thrombi

↓

On fusion soon becomes a homogenous mass

↓

Fibrin is seldom observed in rapidly flowing blood
(Sine, it takes 4 min, so, thromboplastin and fibrinogen swept away)

↓

Hence, heart and major arteries pale thrombus seen

↓

But, in veins having slow moving stream

↓

Fibrin attached to platelet

↓

RBCs and WBCs are entrapped in thrombus

↓

So closely resemble blood clot

↓

Red thrombus

↓

Thrombus gradually increase in size and
Obstruct blood flow

↓

Again favours fibrin formation

↓

Enlarged thrombus occlude the blood vessel

↓

Flow of blood ceases

↓

Stagnant column on either side and expand

Morphology of thrombus

1. Aortic or cardiac thrombi: Typically non-occlusive (Mural) as a result of rapid and high volume flow
2. Smaller artery: Occlusive; Above two thrombi begin at the site of endothelial injury or turbulence (vessel at bifurcation)
3. Venous thrombi: Occlusive; Characteristically at site of stasis

Platelet activators

These are
Thrombin, ADP and TxA2

↓

Bind to receptors
Inhibits adenyl cyclase enzyme

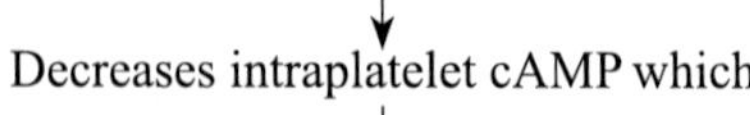

Decreases intraplatelet cAMP which

↓

Platelet aggregation by initiating interaction between
Platelet membrane glycoprotein acceptors and plasma-platelet derived fibrinogen

↓

Prostacyclin, a potent anticoagulant

↓

Activates adenyl cyclase

↓

Increases cAMP

↓

Reduces platelet aggregation by inhibiting function of
Fibrinogen-binding receptors

Endothelial Cell Functions and Responses in Homeostasis and Disease

Fluid distribution and blood flow

Semipermeable membrane for fluid distribution

- Interendothelial junctions

Vasodilation

- Nitric oxide
- Prostacyclin (PGI2)
- Endothelial-derived hyperpolarizing factor
- C-type natriuretic peptide

Vasoconstriction

- Endothelin
- Reactive oxygen species
- Angiotensin II
- Products of prostaglandin H2 (e.g. thromboxane A2)

Hemostasis

Antihemostatic substances

- PGI2
- Endothelial cell protein C receptor
- Tissue factor pathway inhibitor (TFPI)
- Tissue plasminogen activator (tPA)
- Heparan sulfate
- Adenosine diphosphatase (ADPase) and adenosine
- triphosphatase (ATPase)
- Protein S
- Thrombomodulin

Prohemostatic substances

- von Willebrand factor
- Tissue factor (TF) (factor III)
- Plasminogen activator inhibitor-1 (PAl-1)
- Protease-activated receptors (PARs)

Classification of Thrombi

Based on location within blood vascular system

1) Cardiac Thrombi

Heart wall (**Mural thrombus**)

Valves (**Valvular thrombus)**

Mural Thrombus : Seen on the wall of left auricle

Bovines - Black quarter - Caused by *Clostridium chauvoei*

Valvular Thrombus: Pigs – *Streptococcus pyogenes*

- Erysipelothrix rhusiopathiae

Cattle – *Cornybacterium pyogenes*

Horses – *Streptococcus equi*

Ball Thrombus : Seen in auricle

Unattached

Large

Cause valvular obstruction

2) Arterial Thrombi

Located with arteries

Common in domestic animals

Horses: *Strongylus vulgaris* larvae in anterior mesenteric artery

Dogs: *Spirocerca lupiin* aorta

Cattle: *Onchocerca armillata* in aorta

3) VENOUS THROMBI

Phlebothromobosis

Common in bed ridden patients

Rate in animals

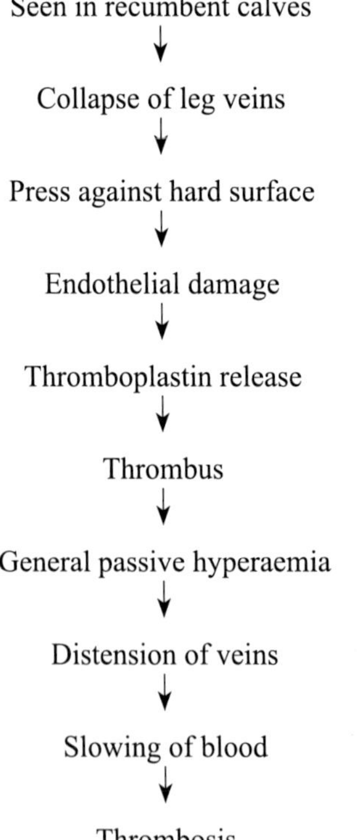

Locations

Human - Femoral, popliteal, iliac veins

Animals - Nasal vascular sinuses – Cow, horses

- Veins of broad ligament – Cow

- Scrotal plexus – Horses

4) Capillary Thrombi

Seen in inflammation

Injury to endothelium

5) Lymphatic Thrombi

Seen in lymphatics draining inflammation area

Beneficial

Classification Based in Location within Heart or Blood Vessels

1) **Mural thrombi**

   Attached to wall of heart / blood vessel

2) **Valuvlar thrombi** attached to valves

3) **Lateral thrombi**

   Attached to one side of blood vessel

4) **Occlusive thrombi**

   Attached to entire circumference of vessel

5) **Saddle thrombi**

   Site of bifurcation of blood vessel

6) **Canalised thrombi**

   New blood channel is formed through clot.

Classification Based on Infectious Agent

1. **Septic thrombi** - contains bacteria
2. **Aseptic thrombi** - Without bacteria / parasites
3. **Parasitic thrombi** - *Strongylus vulgaris* (Horses)

   Dirofilaria immitis (Dogs)

Classification Based on Color of Thrombi

1. **Pale / White Thrombi** - Platelets, seen in heart / aorta
2. **Red Thrombi** - Platelets / fibrin, RBCs, WBCs, seen in veins
3. **Mixed Thrombi** - White and red color

   *Most common

   *White – Rapid blood flow

   *Red – slow blood flow
4. **Laminated thrombi**
5. **Mixed thrombi**

   Excessive exercise - increase blood flow to legs – White thrombus

   Rest- increase blood flow to legs - Red Thrombus There will be alternate red and white thrombus

Fate of Thrombus

Propagation :Enlargement - obstruction of vessel

Contraction : Shrinkage of thrombus fibrous scar

Embolus : Carried to other sites;

Dangerous infarction

Enzymes from WBCs / platelets

Digest thrombi

Fragments emboli

Abscessation : Pyogenic bacteria in thrombus

Bacterial emboli

Resolution : Fibrinolysis

Fresh thrombus - Complete digestion

Old thrombus - incomplete digestion

Organization & Canalization

Significance & Results

1) Negligible effects - Jugular vein; carotid arteries
2) Beneficial effects - Control of haemorrhages
3) Harmful effects - Vessel without collateral circulation
   - Infarction
   - Embolism
   - Passive hyperemia
   - Lymphoedema
   - Aneurysm – *Strongylus vulgaris*
   - Gangrene – intestinal thrombus
   - Colic, lameness
   - Septicaemia / Death

Difference between thrombus and postmortem clot

Character	Thrombus	Post Mortem Clot
• Size	Fills vessels	Smaller than vessel
• Consistency	Dry, friable	Smooth / glistening
• Color	White, red, mixed	Red / yellow
• Attachment	Yes	No
• Endothelium	Damaged	Undamaged
• Composition	Platelets	Fibrin
• Rapidity of blood flow	Formed in flowing stream	Stagnant stream
• Animal	Living	Dead
• Organization	Yes	No
• Structure	Laminated (Line of Zahn)	Homogenous

Embolism

An **embolus** is any foreign body floating in blood. The process is called **embolism.**

Location of Emboli

• Artery / venous / capillaries / lymphatics

In domestic animals emboli always occur in arteries.

In human, venous embolism is common.

Thrombus in leg vein may form emboli to reach large blood vessel, right side heart and pulmonary artery embolism.

Types/causes of Emboli

1. Thrombotic Emboli : Thrombo embolism - arteries (Thrombi detach to form emboli)

Heart - vegetations

Parasitic; atherosclerotic; bacteria

2. Bacterial Emboli : Septicaemia

3. Parasitic Emboli ; *Dirofilaria immitis* - Pulmonary artery - Dog

Schistosomes - Portal; Mesenteric; Nasal

Blood vessels

Trypanasomes - Tartar emetic rapidly

↓

Kills large number of organism

↓

Filarial - Lymphatics

Emboli in brain

↓

Death

4. Neoplastic Emboli : Clumps of tumour cells in circulation producing metastatic tumours

5. Fibrin : Blood transfusion when blood is improperly defibrinated / inadequate anticoagulants

6. Fat Emboli : Fracture of long bones

↓

Fatty marrow

↓

Lungs

↓

Sudden death

"Fat Embolism Syndrome'

(Acute respiratory symptoms, tachycardia, neurological symptoms)

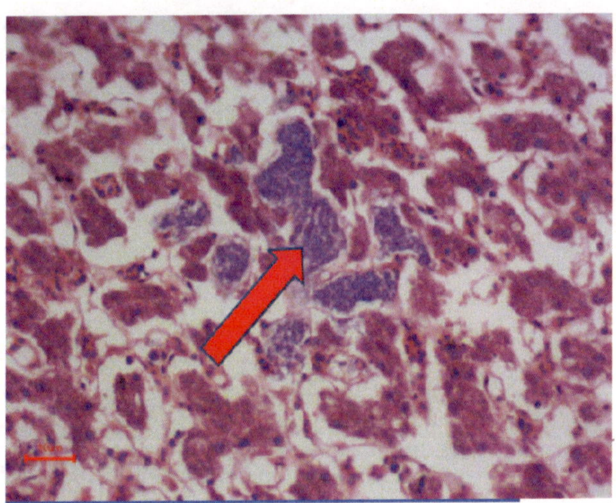

Bacterial emboli (Arrow)

7. Air or Gas Emboli

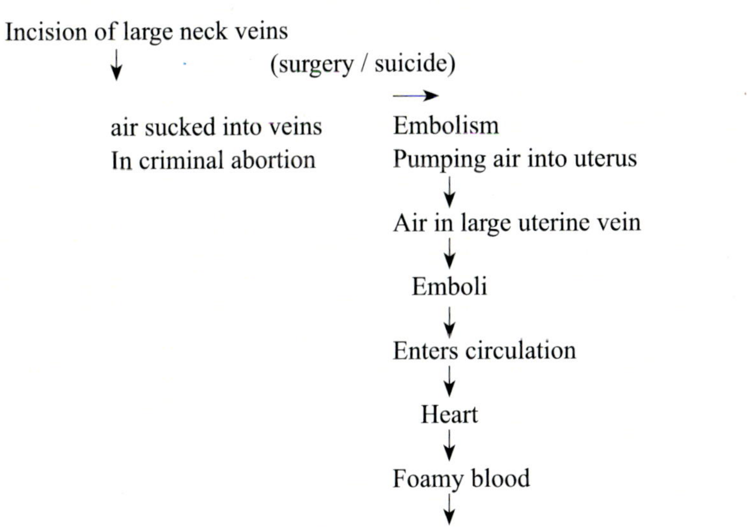

8. Caisson's Disease

Humans

A type of gas embolism

Sudden change in atmospheric pressure

- Under water construction workers
- Deep sea / scuba divers

Unpressurised aircrafts ascends rapidly

Under water construction worker?

Increase air pressure within under water compartment to compensate

↓

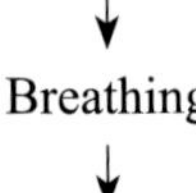

Breathing

↓

Increase air dissolve in blood, tissue, fluid and fat

↓

It the worker surfaces suddenly i.e decompresses

↓

Dissolved gases come OUT as bubbles (O_2 CO_2, N_2)

↓

O_2 and CO_2 are soluble and cause no harm; Nitrogen which is insoluble form

↓

Cause AIR embolism (brain, heart etc)

"Caisson" means - water tight chamber used underwater

The disease is also called as "Bends" in humans, Since, the patients is in bend condition - severe cramping pain

9. Clumps of Normal Body Cells

Occurs when tissue / organ is damaged

Amniotic Fluid Embolism

Complication of labour

Infusion of amniotic fluid (Epithelial cells, fat, mucin, meconium)

↓

Maternal circulation

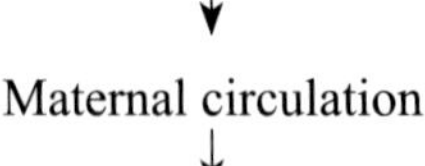

↓

Due to tear in placental membrane or rupture of uterine veins

↓

Maternal mortality

(Respiratory distress; cyanosis, shock, convulsions, coma, death)

Rare in domestic animals - due to anatomical differences in placental / uterine structures

10. Paradoxical Emboli

Emboli that pass directly from the right auricle into the left auricle through patent foramen ovale thereby emboli originating from vein will be lodged in systemic vessels instead of being in pulmonary vessels.

Significance / Result of Embolism

Character of emboli

Size - large emboli → large blood vessel blocked Septic / aseptic – new foci of infection Neoplasms – metastasis

Number of emboli- Increased sites of obstruction

Organs involved

Liver / Lung / muscle - Large blood supply- very little effect

Heart / Kidney / Spleen - no collateral circulation- Impact

Infarction

An infarct is an area of coagulative necrosis results due to sudden blockage of an end artery which has no collateral circulation.

Causes

- Thrombus / embolus
- Pressure on the vessel wall causing ischaemia
- Ligatures
- Decubitus ulcers
- Torniquets
- Tumours
- Cysts / abscess

Volvulus / intussusception of intestine

Contraction of vessel wall

Ergot poisoning

↓

Smooth muscle contraction

↓

Narrowing of blood vessel
↓
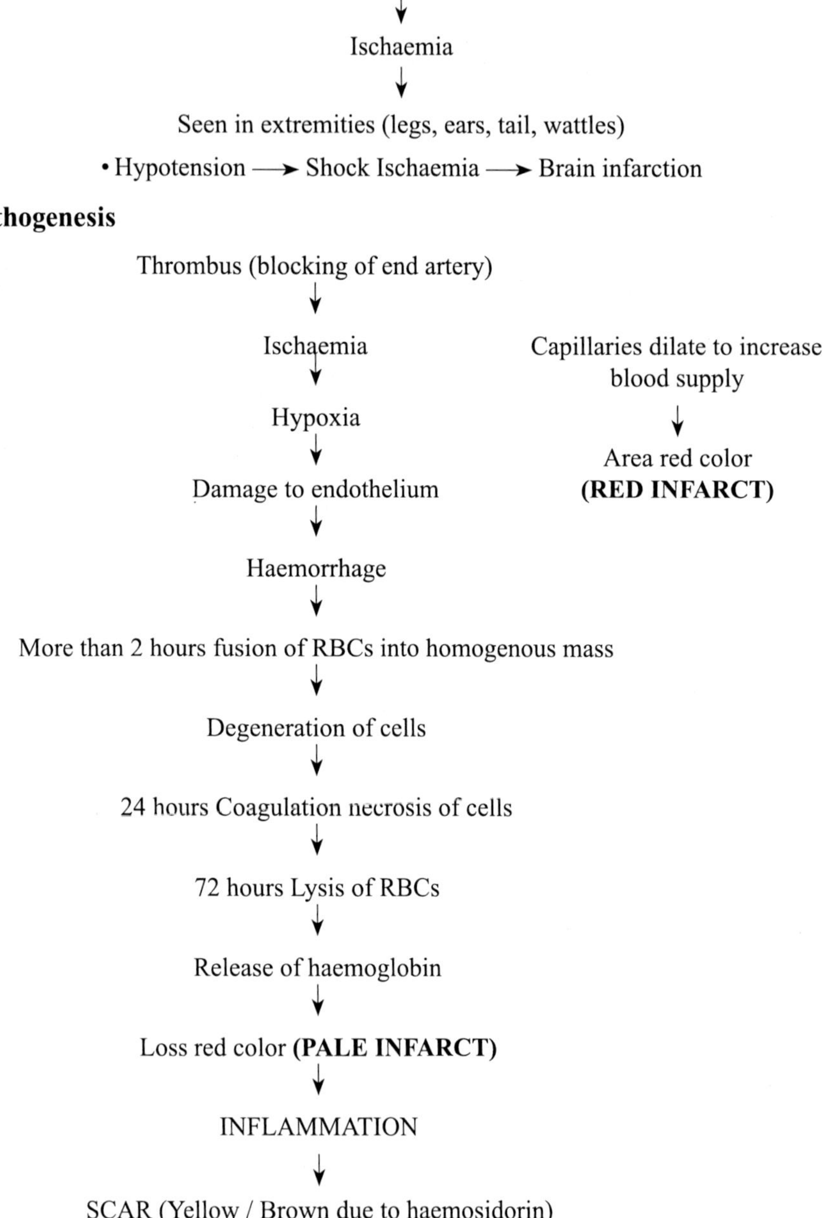

Macroscopical Appearances

Red or pale in color

Cone shaped – apex of cone is at the point of obstruction of vessel

– base towards periphery

Infarcts of Kidneys

- Common in cows and pigs
- Yellow or pale
- Wedge shaped – seen in cortex
- Apex at arcuate arteries
- Base at capsular end of cortex
- No capsular necrosis
- Appears as healed, depressed areas

Causes

Cardiac vegetations – *Corynebacterium pyogenes*, Streptococci

Cows – very common – emboli of uterine vein after parturition

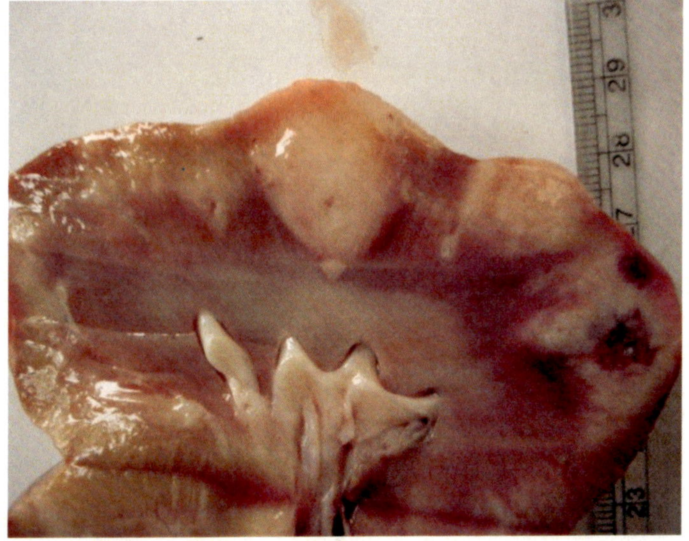

Renal Infarct-Dog-Wedge/Cone shaped

2. Infarcts of Spleen

- Pale or red color
- Seen in borders
- But in dogs, it is band -like
- Due to cardiac thrombi

3. Infarction of Intestines

Common in horses - anterior mesenteric artery (Strongyle worms}

Whole surface of bowel is affected

Red in color

Causes

Volvulus, intussusception, strangulation

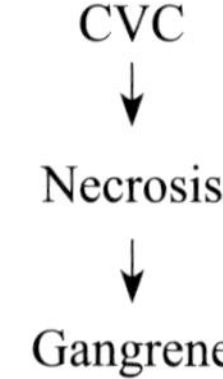

Sequelae

- Fatal
- Toxaemia
- Shock
- Peritonitis

4. Infarction of Brain

Common in man due to arteriosclerosis

Animals - Dogs - automobile accidents

↓

Cerebral infarction

↓

Softening ⟶ Myelin engulfed by microglia -

"Compound Granular Corpuscles"

↓

Organization or cyst formation (neuroglial cells)

Cyst with yellow fluid **"Apoplectic Cysts"**

5. Infarcts of Heart

Common in man due to arteriosclerosis

Not seen in animals

Red or pale

Healed infarcts - Scar

Sequalae of cardiac infarcts – **Myomalacia cardis**

6. Infarcts of Liver

- Tumours
- Thrombus due to *Clostridium hemolyticum* in bovines
- Red in colour

7. Infarcts of Lungs

Common

Cone shaped

Red color

Causes

Emboli from

- Cows – Uterine veins and posterior vena cava (Abscess)
- Horses – Mesenteric veins
- Pigs – Pulmonary veins (Hog cholera)
- Hypostatic congestion
- Chronic venous congestion

Cattle & Sheep – Pasteurella infection → Pulmonary infarction (Haemorrhagic septicaemia)

Sequelae of Infarcts

- Organization and scar formation
- Gangrene
- Death (Brain, heart, intestine) – SHOCK/ Toxaemia/ Septicaemia

Shock "*Cardiovascular collapse*"

A common grave medical emergency characterized by a reduction in effective circulating blood volume and in the blood pressure.

- Shock (cardiovascular collapse) is a circulatory dishomeostasis associated with loss of circulating blood volume and reduced output and or inappropriate peripheral vascular resistance.
- Although causes of shock can be diverse the underlying cause of shock are relatively stereotyped **i.e. hypoperfusion.**

Causes of Shock

- Trauma / burns
- Profuse haemorrhage
- Bacterial septicaemia
- Myocardial infarction (man)
- Pulmonary embolism (man)
- Psychic stimuli (man)
- Crushing (Tissue trauma) injuries (automobile accidents) in dogs
- Cold, exhaustion, depression, general anaesthesia in animals

Classification of Shock

- **Primary**
- **Secondary**

Primary (Syncope, fainting) shock

Appears immediately after extensive injury

Nervous stimuli in which widespread paralysis of capillaries occurs

Animals

Rough handling of animals

Undue manipulation of intestine in abdominal surgery

Humans

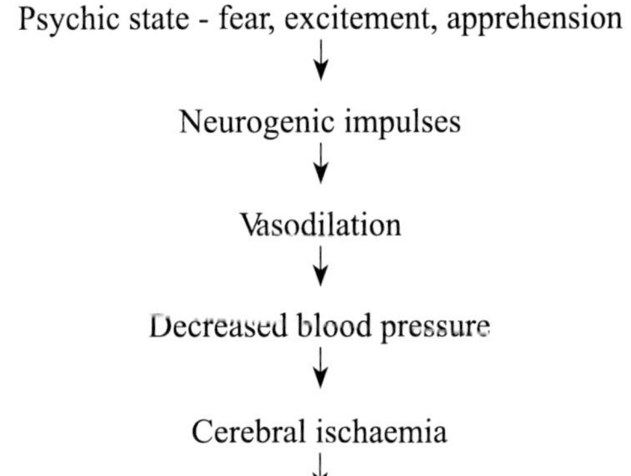

↓

Loss of consciousness (Pallid face, slow breathing, feeble pulse) Transient/ Patient recovers with rest,

Secondary Shock

It is fatal

Disproportion in blood volume and volume of blood vascular space

↓

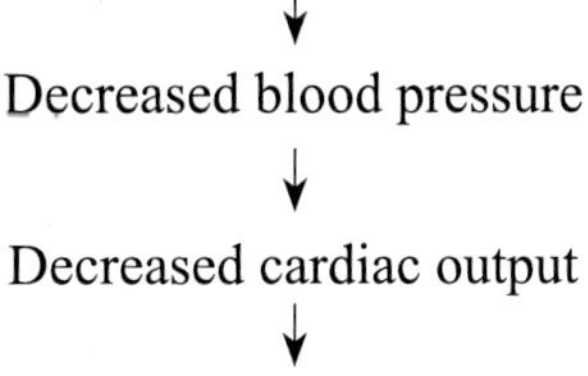

↓

Reflex sympathetic vasoconstriction (Pallor of skin)

↓

Aldosterone, renin —Angiotensin activated

↓

Renal ischaemia Death

↓

Increased cardiac action, decreased pulse rate

↓

Death

Causes of Shock

1. Reduction in Blood Volume

Loss of blood from injuries (Haemorrhages)

Loss of fluid into injured tissues

- Severe burns
- Crushing injuries Oedema
- Vomition
- Diarrhoea Dehydration
- Sodium deficiency
- Addison's disease Dehydration
- Diabetic coma
- Poisons (Phosgene, mustard gas, ANTU)

2. Capillary Bed Dilation

Decreased cardiac output → decreased blood volume

- Neurogenic stimuli
- Anxiety, fear, pain, bleeding wounds
- Bacterial toxins
- Burns, crushing injuries
- Anoxia

3 Acute Circulatory Failure

Infarction, cardiac tamponade

Pulmonary embolism → No circulation → Shock

Classification Based on Fundamental Underlying Problem

1. Cardiogenic shock
2. Hypovolemic shock
3. Blood maldistribution shock
4. Septic shock

5. Anaphylactic shock
6. Neurogenic shock

1. Cardiogenic shock results from failure of heart to adequately pump blood.

This occurs due to

- Myocardial infarction
- Ventricular tachycardia
- Fibrillation or other arrhythmia
- Dilating and cardiac myopathy
- Obstruction of blood flow from the heart

  e.g. Pulmonary embolism and pulmonary or aortic stenosis
- Other cardiac dysfunction
- Unsuccessful compensation leads to stagnation of blood and progressive tissue hypo perfusion.

2. Hypovolemic shock arises from reduced circulatory blood volume due to blood loss caused by haemorrhage of fluid loss secondary to vomiting, diarrhoea or burns

- This leads to decreased vascular permeability and tissue hypoperfusion.
- Immediate compensatory mechanisms to increase vascular pressure
- Vasoconstriction and fluid movement into plasma.
- Loss of about 10% blood volume can occur without consequence, but when blood loss approaches 35-45% blood pressue and cardiac output can fall dramatically.

3. Blood maldistribution shock is characterized by decreased peripheral vascular resistance and pooling of blood in peripheral tissue.

- The systemic vascular dilatation results may dramtically increase microvascular area and although the blood volume is normal.
- The effective circulating blood volume is decreased.

4. Septic Shock

- Microthrombosis is common.
- Common type of shock associated with blood maldistribution.
- Here components of bacteria or fungi (endotoxin, a lipopolysaccharide (LPS) within the cell wall of gram negative bacteria) which are released from degenerating bacteria is potent stimulus and causes for septic shock.

5. Anaphylactic shock

It is generalized type I hypersensitivity.

Causes

Exposure to

- Insect bites
- Plant poisons
- Drugs
- Vaccine
- Interaction of an inciting substance with gE and mast cell results in mast cell degranulation, release of histamine and systemic vascular dilatation, increased vascular permeability and tissue hypoperfusion.

6. Neurogenic shock

Causes

- Trauma (particularly of nervous system)
- Electrocution (Lightning stroke)
- Fear
- Emotional stress
- Here autonomic discharge that results in peripheral dilatation followed by venous pooling of blood and tissue hypoperfusion. When compared to anaphylactic and endotoxic shock wherein cytokines play a major role in initial peripheral vascular dilatation. In neurogenic shock autonomic discharges that result in peripheral vasodilatation, venous stasis and tissue hypoperfusion

Three Major types of shock

Type of shock	Clinical Example	Principal Mechanisms
Cardiogenic	Myocardial infarction Ventricular rupture Arrhythmia Cardiac tamponade Pulmonary embolism	Failure of myocardial pump resulting from intrinsic myocardial damage, extrinsic compression, or obstruction to outflow
Hypovolemic	Fluid loss (e.g. hemorrhage, vomiting , diarrhea, burns or trauma)	Inadequte blood or plasma volume
Shock associated with systemic inflammation	Overwhelming microbial infections (bacterial and fungal) Superantigens (e.g toxic shock syndrome) Trau- ma, burns, pancreatitis	Activation of cytokine cascades, peripheral vasodilation and pooling of blood: endothelial activation / injury; leukocyte induced damage, disseminated intravasuclar coagulation

Important Pathways in Septic Shock

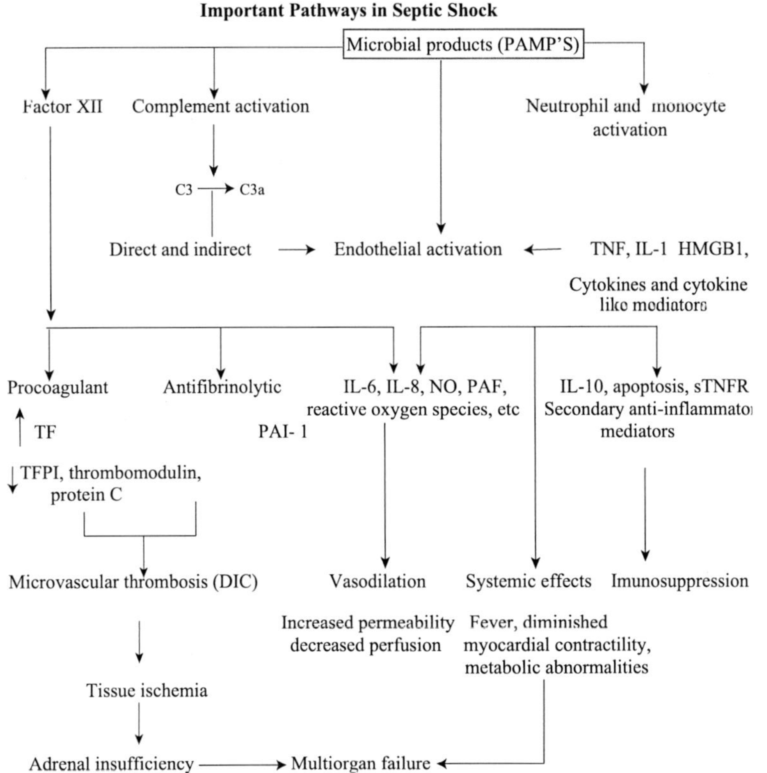

Microbial products: Pathogen associated molecular patterns (PAMPS) DIC Disseminated vascular coagulation, HMGB1 high mobility group box 1 protein, NO, nitric oxide, PAF, platelet activating factor, PAI-1, Plasminogen activator inhibitor 1 TF, tissue factor, TFPI, tissue factor pathway inhibitor.Plasminogen activator inhibitor 1 TF, tissue factor, TFPI, tissue factor pathway inhibitor.

Septic Shock

- Common type of shock associated with blood maldistribution.
- Here components of bacteria or fungi (endotoxin, a lipopolysaccharide within the cell wall of gram negative bacteria) which are released from degenerating bacteria is potent stimulus and causes for septic shock.

Pathogenesis of Shock

Ischaemic Shock

Septic Shock

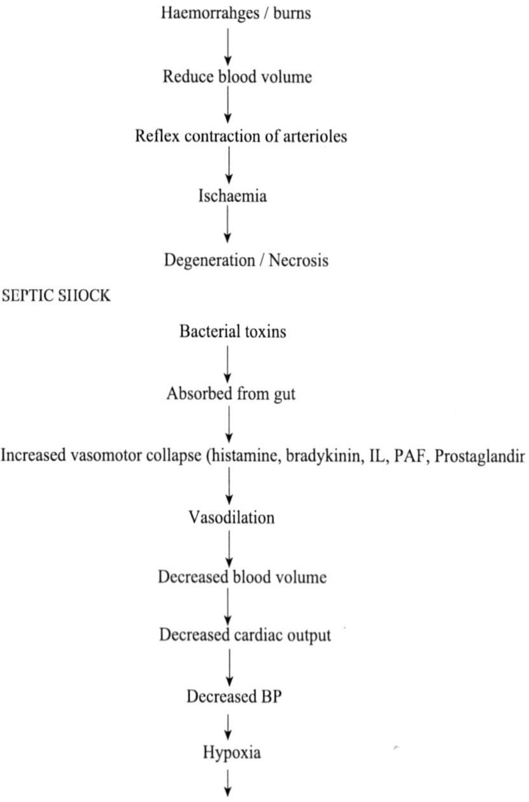

VASOACTIVE PRINCIPLES

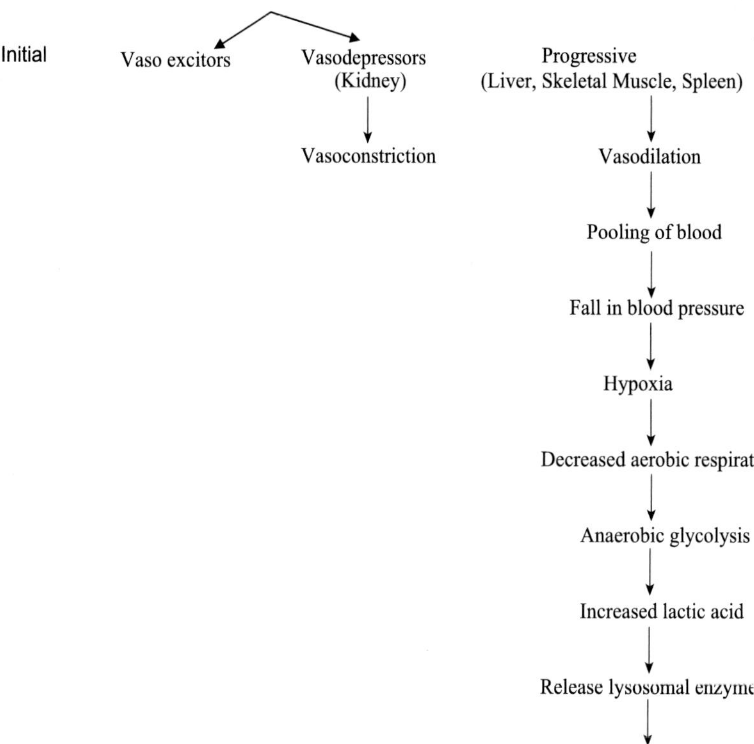

Signs of Shock

- Rapidly progessive
- Lethargy; recumbent; weak pulse rate, hypotension, tachcardia
- Cold extremities (hypovolumic)
- Anxiousness
- Shallow breathing
- Pulmonary rales
- Reduced urine output
- Multiorgan failure with respective clinical signs

Microscopical Appearance

- Depends on nature and severity
- Venules and capillaries engorged with blood (Generalized congestion)
- Pooling of blood
- Fat embolism in lungs – traumatic shock
- Hypoxic injury
- Fatty degeneration and necrosis in liver / heart
- Renal tubular necrosis – casts in tubules
- Gastrointestinal epithelial necrosis
- Adrenal cortex is foamy, due to depletion of cholesterol
- Neurons and cardiomyocytes are highly susceptible
- Pulmonary congestion, oedema and haemorrhages
- Necrosis of alveolar epithelium, fibrinous exudation and hyaline membrane formation
- Cerebral ischemia and oedema
- Intestinal mucosa congested, oedematous and haemorrhagic
- Vascular changes- Disseminated intravascular coagulation
- Changes are reversible except for neuronal and myocytic injury/damage

Significance and Results

- Recovery - on blood transfusion / supportive treatment
- Death - irreversible shock

Renal insufficiency

- Oliguria, anuria, uraemia
- Pigment casts in tubules
- Inflammatory oedema compresses renal parenchyma
- Ischaemia - due to vascular collapse
- Tubular degeneration and necrosis

Cardiac Failure

Cerebral Ischaemia-decreased BP ⟶ Anoxia ⟶ Neuronal degeneration

↓

Encephalomalacia

↓

Death

Pulmonary Infection - Pulmonary oedema Bacterial growth

Stages of shock-Three

1. Non-progressive stage
2. Progressive stage
3. Irreversible stage

1. Non – progressive stage of shock

Compensatory mechanisms counteract.

i. Reduced functional blood volume

ii. Decreased vascular pressure (baroceptors respond)-increased sympathetic nerve stimulation and epinephrine /norepinephrine release: which increase cardiac output and peripheral resistance through vasoconstriction; ADH and angiotensin-II; endothelin, cold, increase oxygen or decreased CO_2 also vasoconstrictive.

iii. Reduced plasma volume stimulates

- ADH release
- Water retention
- Activates angiotensin-II production by renin-angiotensin system → results in aldosterone release and sodium retention.

iv. Consequences: increased heart rate, cardiac output and increased blood pressure

v. In mild cases these mechanisms help to compensate and reverse to normal homeostasis.

2. Progressive stage of shock

Severe as prolonged hypovolemia or cardiac damage occurs. Compensatory mechanism become inadequate and shock enters progressive stage.

- Blood pooling, tissue hypoperfusion and progressive cell injury
- Cellular and systemic lactic acidosis seen aerorbic (Kreb's cycle) metabolism switched to anaerobic and over production of lactic acid from pyruvate and depletion of ATP
- Atreolar relaxation and dilatation; metabolic products like adenosine and potassium, increased local osmolarity, hypoxia and increased CO_2.
- Septic shock: The above events are exacerbated with cytokines and inflammatory mediators.
- Cardiogenic and hypovolemic shock-dormant vascular bed opened and stagnation of blood occurs.
- Decreased energy and hypoxia resulted in necrosis with release of lysosomal enzymes
- Dramatic accumulation of mediators occurs, mainly histamine, kinins, PAE, complement fragment, cytokine-TNF, IL-1, 8; due to inappropriate systemic inflammation and systemic activation of complement, coagulation, fibrinolysis and kinin system.

3. Irreversible stage of shock

Exact time of entry to this stage is not known.

Attributed to anaerobic metabolism, cellular acidosis
Energy metabolism is affected

↓

Ischemic tissue-inflammatory mediators accumulate

↓

Override central vasoconstriction mechanism

↓

Vasodilatation

↓

Fall in peripheral blood pressure

↓

Multiorgan failure (liver, kidney, intestine and heart)
One organ failure contributes to affection of others

↓

DIC (Disseminated Intravascular Coagulation)
End point of irreversible shock

Profound and paradoxical dysfunction of haemostasis

↓

Septic shock

↓

Endotoxin LPS (Lipopolysaccharide)-Gram -ve organism
(most common cause)

↓

Enter bowel

↓

LPS produced

↓

Reach liver, spleen, alveoli leukocytes through circulation-entry into monocytes-macrophage system (MMs)

↓

Shwartzman reaction (experimental model)
Hypersensitive to LPS

↓

Priming i/v LPS (macrophage stimulation by IFN-gamma of lymphocytes)
and
proinflammatory cytokine, IL-12, IFN-gamma

↓

24h challenge i/v with LPS

↓

Primed macrophages produced high TNF (Proinflammatory cytokine)
particularly

↓

Stages of shock

1. Early shock-non progres- sive	**2. Progressive shock**	**3. Irreversible shock**
Only a small decrease in blood volume Neurohormonal mechanism (constriction of atreolar bed+ increase heart rate etc) ↓ Maintain BP and cardiac output vasoconstriction responsible for coolness and paleness	Appears with persistence of shock ↓ cardiac output and BP ↓ Vital organs experience significant hypoxia ↓ Revert to anaerobic gly-colysis ↓ Metabolic lactic acidosis ↓ Abnormal rapidity respira-tion (tachypnoea Marked reduction in urinary output-oliguria) marked deterioration of patient	Even treatment does not stop the deteriorating condition of the patient ↓ Transition from reversible to irreversible ↓ Progressive decreased cardiac output and fallen P ↓ Decreased flow to brain heart and kidney ↓ with ischemic cell death ↓ Coma renal failure, ure-mia and death

Morphology of Shock

Hypoxic Cell Injury

Brain – Neurons – reversible cell injury

Irreversible cell injury (ischaemic encephalopathy)

Heart – Subpericardial / Subendocardial haemorrhages and necrosis

Kidneys – Acute tubular epithelial cell necrosis

Lungs – Resistant to hypoxic cell injury

– Not affected in hypovolemic shock

– But changes seen in endotoxic or neurogenic shock

GIT – Patchy mucosal haemorrhages "Haemorrhagic enteropathy"

Liver – Fatty changes / central necrosis

4

Amyloidosis and Storage Diseases (Glycogen, fat and lysosomal)

Amyloid

- Amyloid (G. Amylon; Amyl(o) - STARCH) means starch-like.
- Amyloid is a pathologic glycoprotein deposited in the extracellular spaces and forms fibrils on polymerization.

Histological characteristics

- Amyloid is specially stained with Congo Red.
- Under polarized light, green birefringence is noticed because of alignment of fibrils.
- Amyloid fibrils are 7.5 to 10 nm in diameter, rigid, non-branching hollow-cored tubules of unknown length.
- **β-pleated** sheet configuration is seen in X-ray diffraction.
- The P-component which is a glycosa-amino-glycan (GAG) facilitates polymerization of amyloid.
- The GAG makes the amyloid to stain with iodine.
- The amyloid is resistant to enzymatic digestion and progressively accumulated in tissues until the underlying disease process persists.

Types/Sources of amyloid

Amyloid associated (AA)

- It occurs in chronic diseases and septic conditions. Precursor is serum amyloid associated protein (SAA).

Amyloid light-chain (AL)

- It is produced in plasmacytoma and the precursor is immunoglobulin light-chain.
- The AL occurs in pulmonary arteries and derived from apolipoprotein AL.
- IAPP is associated with pancreatic islets and derived from **islet amyloid polypeptide.**
- In the brain of aged animals, beta amyloid protein is produced from beta amyloid precursor protein.

Amyloidosis

- It is an immunological disorder in which homogeneous, translucent amyloid substance is deposited between capillary endothelium and adjacent cells.

Pathogenesis

- The main event occurring in amyloidosis is the deposition of amyloid fibrils due to abnormality of protein processing.
- The sources of amyloid may be acute phase proteins, immunoglobulins and endocrine secretes.
- The abnormal variant proteins are continuously incorporated to form fibrils.
- The preamyloid substances are soluble and synthesized in the cytoplasm and deposited in the extracellular spaces.
- The amyloid forms a β-pleated sheet despite their chemical heterogeneity.
- This makes the fibril resistant to digestion by macrophages and phagocytic cells and hence accumulates in tissues.
- The fibrils may disappear following the removal of cause. Splenic active macrophages remove the amyloid fibrils, but not in the kidneys.
- The amyloid, deposited around the blood vessels is more dangerous.

Effects are

- Pressure atrophy of the adjacent cells from ischaemic anoxia results in degeneration and necrosis.

- Due to interference with gaseous exchange, nutrition supply and waste products removal affected due to stenotic vessels.
- Degeneration and necrosis of cells will occur

Types of Amyloidosis

1. Primary Amyloidosis

2. Secondary Amyloidosis

1. Primary Amyloidosis

- It results from antigen-antibody reaction and deposition of its precipitates.
- The condition is not associated with any disease. It is occurs in e.g. repeated exposure to antigens as in antisera and antitoxin production in horses and B cell dyscrasia (plasmacytoma) in humans in which immunoglobin light chain deposition occurs.
- The soluble immunoglobulin becomes insoluble with defective degradation

2.Secondary Amyloidosis

- The condition may be associated with chronic diseases like tuberculosis, septic conditions and neoplasia.
- The serum amyloid associated proteins (SAA) increase and converted to insoluble amyloid associated substances. This occurs in two phases.
- In the **initial preamyloid phase**, there is accumulation of reticular cells and macrophages in the spleen and other lymphoid tissue with consequent rise in plasma SAAs and globulins.
- Probably, the cytokines and interleukin-1 from macrophages stimulate the liver to synthesize SAAs.
- During the second phase, known as **amyloid phase**, PAS staining cells, amyloid deposition and fall in the SAAs level are found.
- Animals affected are dogs, cattle, horses and chickens. Spleen, liver, kidney, lymph node and adrenals are commonly affected.

Gross Pathology

- The amyloid deposition may be diffuse or focal. The amyloid is deposited around the central artery of splenic follicles

- It forms sheet - like deposits which is referred as **bacon spleen.**
- It may protrude resembling - like a grain of sago known as **sago spleen**.
- The organ is waxy (Previously called as waxy degeneration) in consistency and the cut surface is grayish.
- Splenic corpuscles become large, gray and translucent.
- Enlargement of liver with rounded edges, doughy consistency, pits on pressure and ruptures easily because of its friable nature.
- In renal amyloidosis, the organ is swollen, mottled, pale and yellow to orange in colour

Effects of Amyloidosis

- Hypovolemic or haemorrhagic shock may occur following hepatic rupture.
- The deposition of amyloid is found between the endothelium of sinusoids and cords of hepatic cells.

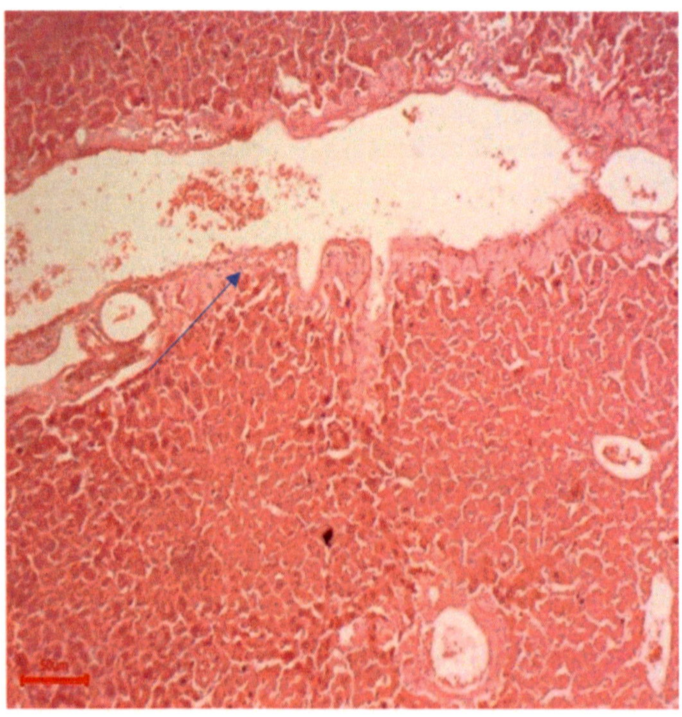

Liver-Extracellular amyloidosis (Arrow)

- Hepatocellular atrophy occurs from pressure and nutritional deficiency.
- In renal amyloidosis, amyloid deposition occurs between capillary endothelium and epithelium of glomeruli interfering with glomerular circulation.
- The enlargement and ischaemic anoxia leads to tubular epithelial cell degeneration and necrosis, marked proteinuria, nephrotic syndrome, uremia and death.
- In pancreatic amyloidosis, the deposition of amyloid is found between the capillary and islet cells leading to islet cell destruction and development of Diabetes mellitus.
- Blindness may be encountered in horses with conjuctival amyloid deposition.

Glycogen Overload

- It is excessive intracellular accumulation of glycogen with derangement in glucose or glycogen metabolism. The condition is not a significant entity in animals as compared to humans. Glycogen overload may be encountered in:
- Neutrophils in inflammation
- Fast growing neoplastic cells
- Necrotic areas
- Diabetes mellitus
- Liver of young and growing animals
- Well-fed animals

Glycogen Storage Diseases (Glycogenoses)

- The cells may accumulate abnormal amount of glycogen in the cytoplasm. The cells are swollen with foamy cytoplasm. The condition is not common in animals. It may be associated with prolonged hyperglycaemia and there may be lack of enzymes that metabolize carbohydrates. It is a group of diseases in which two forms are recognized in animals.
- Type II or Pompe's disease: There is deficiency of lysosomal α-glucosidase with accumulation of glycogen in the lysosome of brain, muscle and liver. This condition is seen in cattle, dogs, cats and sheep.

- Type III or Cori-Forbes' disease: There is deficiency of amylo-1,6-glucosidase which converts glycogen to glucose. Hence, glycogen is stored in the cytoplasm of liver, heart, skeletal and smooth muscle and nerve cells. This condition is reported in dogs and cats.

Type Ia (von Gierke disease in humans): There is deficiency of glucose-6-phosphatase that catalyses hydrolysis of glucose-6-phosphate to glucose and phosphate. Affected pups show tremors, weakness and neurological signs due to hypoglycaemia and growth retardation and progressive hepatomegaly are found as they develop. Massively enlarged hepatocytes show vacuolations with aggregation

Fatty Changes (Hepatic Lipidosis)

It is the accumulation of triglycerides or true fats and cholesterol in the cytoplasm of parenchymatous cells. Lipidosis is more common than other conditions.

Mechanism of Hepatic Lipidosis

- Mobilization of free fatty acids from the gut (Chylomicrons) or adipose tissue
- Mitochondrial injury leading to decreases in β-oxidation of fatty acids to ketones etc. (Hypoxia, toxins)
- Decreased apolipoprotein synthesis e.g. CCl poisoning and aflatoxicosis
- Failure to form lipoproteins
- Failure to release lipoproteins from hepatocytes
- The last two conditions are uncommon.
- Hepatic lipidosis can occur from one or more mechanisms.
- Fatty acid mobilisation from adipose tissue is common in animals following higher energy demand.
- Starvation increases triglyceride mobilisation.
- Protein malnutrition affects apolipoprotein synthesis.
- Chemicals like CCl steatosis. and yellow phosphorous can also induce hepatic

Grossly

- Enlarged, pale to yellow, soft and friable liver is found in moderate to higher grade fatty changes
- Rounded borders
- Upon incision, fat droplets are seen on the blades of knife.
- Tissue may float in the fixatives.

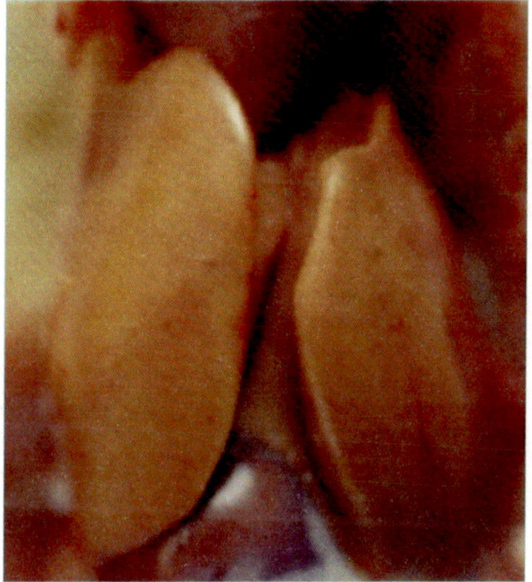

Fatty Liver-Chicken-Yellow discolouration

Microscopically, Hepatocytes show vacuolations which may be small, clear to variable sized and may also form a single large vacuole, pushing the nucleus to a side.

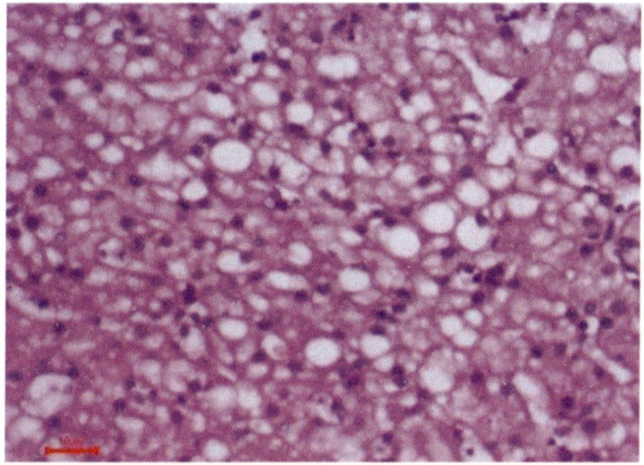

Fatty Changes-Liver-Dog Note: Clear cut vacuoles; nucleus pushed to periphery

- During the processing of fat tissue with xylol clearing, the fat will be dissolved by the xylol and gives vacuolated appearance in the Haematoxylin and eosin stained sections.
- To differentiate from hepatic degeneration, fluid and glycogen accumulation, cryostat sections are used to stain fat.
- Special stans for fats are Sudan III, Sudan black, Scarlet red and Oil Red O.
- Oil Red O stains fat red and is PAS negative, Sudan III and Sudan black imparts black colour and Scarlet red imparts red colour

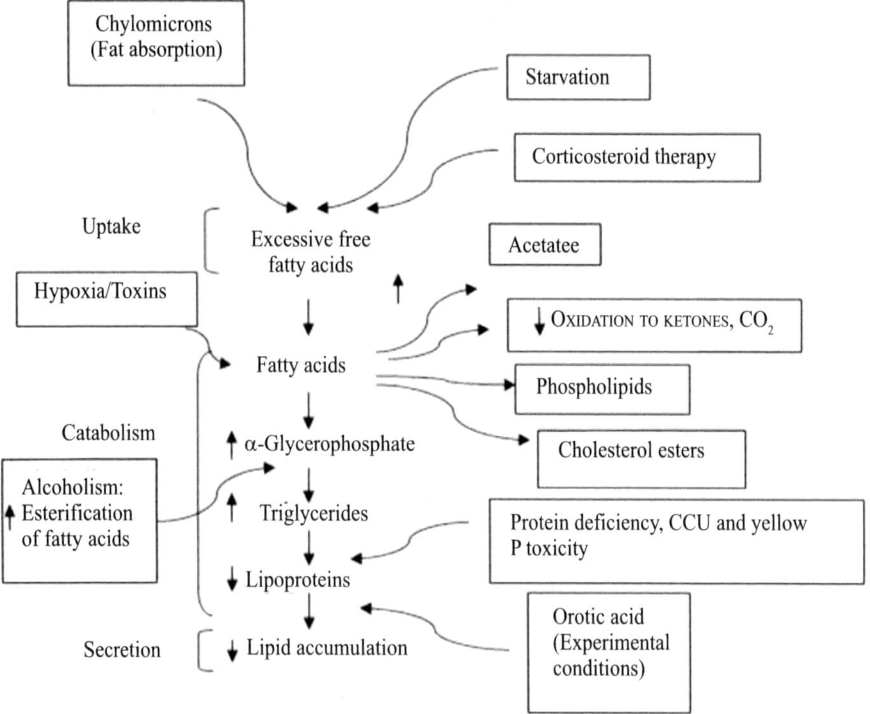

Heat Shock Proteins

Heat shock proteins (HSPs) are intracellular chaperones (Fr. an older woman who looks after a girl, today's context to look after proteins within the cell).

- There are about ten families. e.g. HSP 60, HSP 90 and HSP 70.
- HSPs are not commonly present in blood and body fluids.
- Hence, their presence indicates physical damage.

- These are involved in protein folding, degradation of protein (HSP 70) assembly of protein, thermotolerance, buffering and expression of mutations.
- Stress causes protein aggregation and degradation. e.g. heat, UV radiation, etc
- They also play a role as intracellular chaperones of antigenic peptides. Antigen presenting cells (APC) express receptors that ligate HSP bound antigen peptides.
- HSPs alone or peptide alone is non-immunogenic.
- Combination elicited MHC class I restricted antigen specific CD8 cytotoxic T cell responses (immunity to cancers).

Lysosomal Storage Diseases

These are genetically determined diseases with reduced lysosomal enzyme synthesis and now understood that it may also be caused by other contributory factors like lack of enzyme and substrate activators.

- The lysosomal dysfunction leads to accumulation of normally degraded substrates leading to death of cells.
- The disease kills the developing foetus or may be manifested in neonatal or early life.

Examples

- Lipid storage disease
- Mucopolysaccharidoses
- Mucolipidoses
- Glycogen storage diseases

Lipid Storage Disease

- Lysosomes lacking enzymes that are degrading cellular membranes leading to accumulation of lipid materials in the brain, liver or other organs.
- The central nervous system: a) deficiency of β-galactosidase in the lysosome results in GM1gangliosidosis) deficiency of β-hexosinamidase results in GM2gangliosidosis.

Grossly, atrophy of brain, and rubbery consistency of brain are seen.

Globoid mucodystrophy may occur in later stages with loss of myelin

Microscopically, the neurons are enlarged; cytoplasm is foamy, finely granular and vacuolated with displacement of nuclei.

In GM1gangliosidosis, whorls and laminar arrangements of membranes are seen in the CNS and visceral cells.

Mucopolysaccharidoses

- The defectively degraded glycosaminoglycans (GAG) are stored in the cells that normally degrade them.
- These are genetically determined group of diseases.
- There is lack of specific hydrolases in lysosomes which results in massive accumulations of GAG polymers and formation of giant lysosomes.
- Mucopolysaccharidosis type I, is caused by the absence of a-L-iduronidase in Siamese cats and Plott hound.

Mucolipidoses

- There is genetic deficiency of ganglioside sialidase enzyme and consequent accumulations of glycolipids and GAGs in the form of granulofibrillar vacuoles in hounds.
- The affected animals show deformities of face and bones. Corneas are clouded.
- Abnormally large granules are seen in the leukocytes. Excess GAGs in urine of weaning animals confirms this disease

Naemann-Pick Type-C disease

- There is accumulation of sphingomyelin in lysosomes deficient in sphingomyelinase in dogs and cats.
- The cytoplasm of nerves, hepatocytes and mononuclear cells and phagocytes show vacuolations.

5

Reversible and Irreversible Cell Injury

Causes and Mechanism

I. External Causes/ Extrinsic Causes

1. Physical Causes

1. Trauma by cutting objects and blunt objects
2. Electrical – Lightning, high frequency current
3. Heat -Sun stroke, burns, fever
4. Cold

   Local tissue freezing, cold shock
5. Radiation

   UV / X /cosmic radiations
6. Pressure

   Increased or decreased pressure

2. Chemical Causes

7. Nutritional - Excess / deficiency

   Excess – Hypervitaminoses A and D

   Deficiency –protein, calorie, vitamins and minerals
8. Agrochemicals– nitrates
9. Environmental deficiency Water –dehydration Oxygen –asphyxia

   Sunlight – for vitamin D formation (Hypovitaminosis D)
10. Biological toxins

    Bacterial and fungal toxins

Arthropod and snake venom

Pesticides –organochlorine, organophosphorus compounds etc.

3. Biological Causes

11. Acellular – Viruses, prions
12. Prokaryotes – Bacteria, chlamydia, rickettsia, mycoplasma
13. Eukaryotes – Protozoa, fungi
14. Metazoan parasites – Trematodes, cestodes, nematodes and insects

II. Internal causes/Intrinsic Causes

Genetic Causes– mutation of genes to chromosomal defects

The Common Causes of Cell Injury

1. Hypoxic injury
2. Free radical injury
3. Chemical injury
4. Virus induced injury

1. Events in Ischaemic Cell Injury

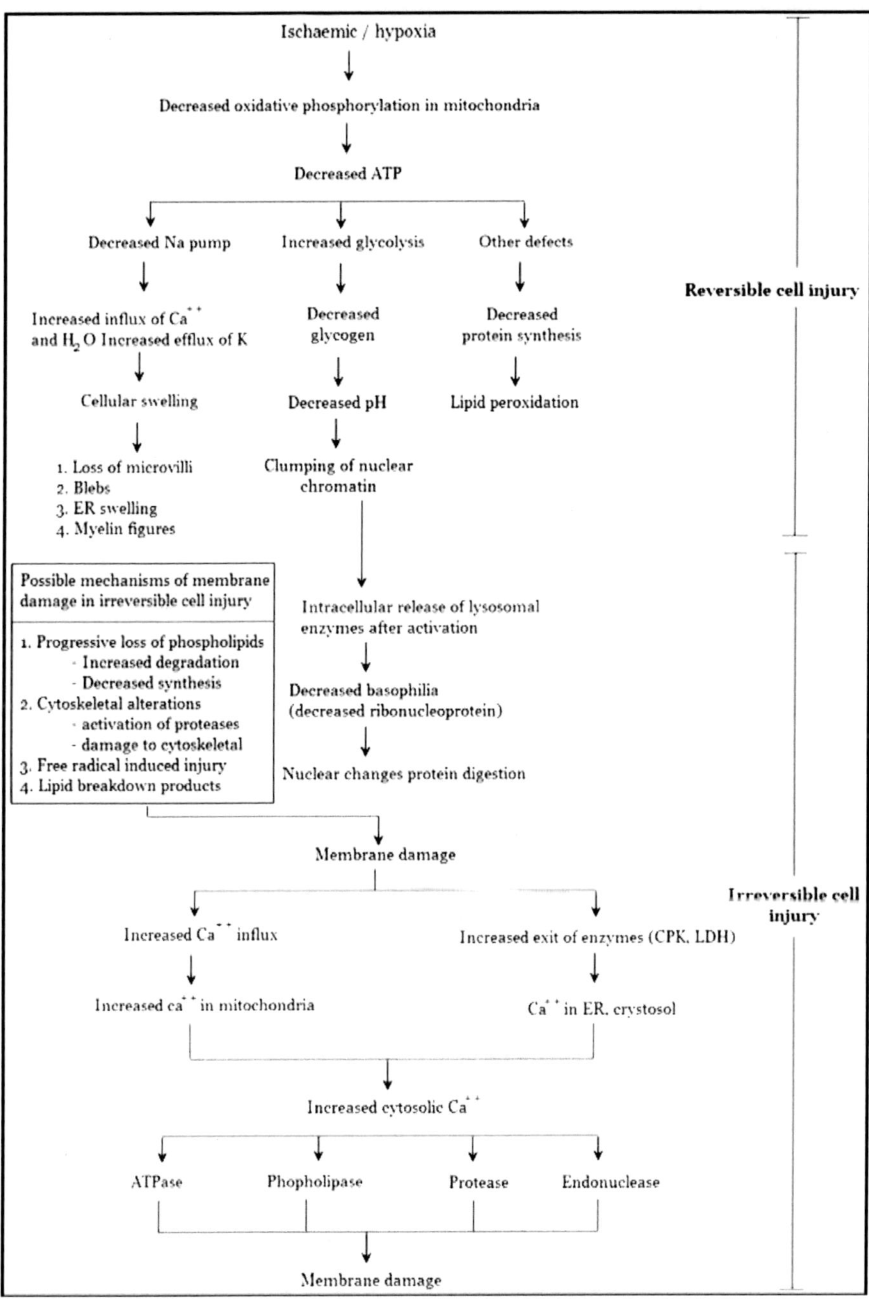

Reversible cell injury is non-lethal and previously referred as degeneration.

Irreversible injury causes necrosis or death of the cells.

The two patterns found in reversible injury are

1. Cellular swelling
2. Fatty change

2. Free Radical Injury

- Free radicals are chemical species that have single unpaired electron in the outer orbit.
- Free radicals are extremely reactive and unstable and enter into reaction with inorganic and organic substances, proteins, lipids or carbohydrates, particularly free radicals react with membrane and nucleic acid.
- They initiate autocatalytic reactions. Free radicals may be initiated in cells with radiant energy (UV /X rays), generation of endogenous oxidative reaction or enzymatic metabolism, exogenous chemicals or drugs e.g. Chloroform, carbon tetrachloride
- The oxygen-derived radicals are superoxide, hydrogen peroxide and hydroxide radicals. These cause lipid peroxidation, protein damage and DNA damage.
- The antioxidants (endogenous or exogenous) are helpful in scavenging the free radicals e.g. Vitamin E, sulphur containing amino acids (cystine, methionine), glutathione and ceruloplasmin.

3. Chemical Injury

- Chemicals can induce cell injury directly by reacting with critical cellular molecules e.g. mercuric chloride poisoning.
- Mercury binds with sulphydryl group and other proteins and cause increased cell membrane permeability and inhibition of ATPase dependant transport or indirectly by converting chemicals which are not biologically active into reactive toxic metabolite that attack target cells.
- Mostly reactive free radicals formed can induce membrane damage and can cause direct injury by covalent binding to membrane lipid and

protein. e.g. Carbon tetrachloride (CCl_4) poisoning.

- Carbon tetrachloride is converted to CCl_3 membrane and generate lipid peroxides.
- The autocatalytic reaction results in membrane damage involving rough endoplasmic reticulum, detachment of ribosomes, reduced protein synthesis and fatty liver due to lack of lipid acceptor protein.
- **Net result : Necrosis and fatty degeneration**
- Lipid peroxidation products can also damage plasma membrane to increase permeability to sodium and water resulting in cell swelling.

4. Virus Induced Cell Injury

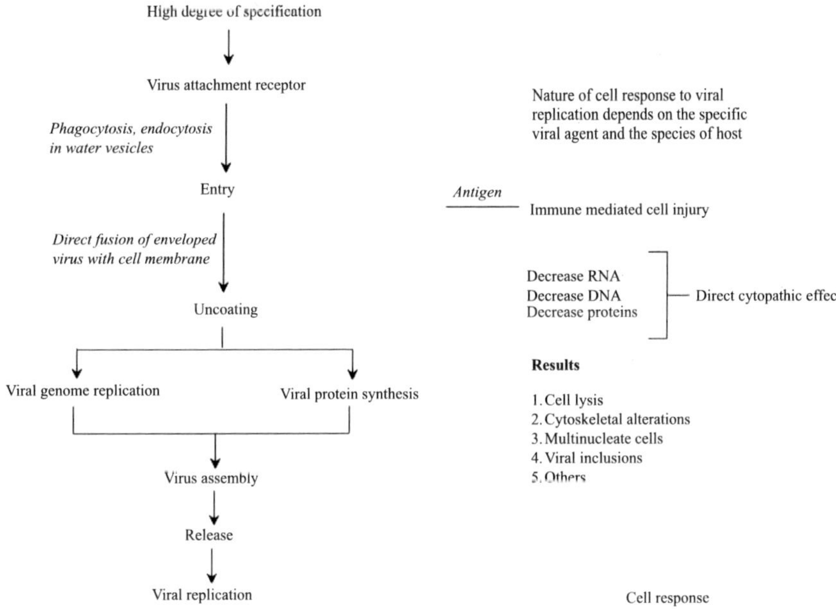

Viruses that induce cellular changes are of two types

Cytolytic / cytopathic viruses which cause various degree of cell injury and cell death.

Oncogenic viruses which stimulate host cell replication and may produce tumours.

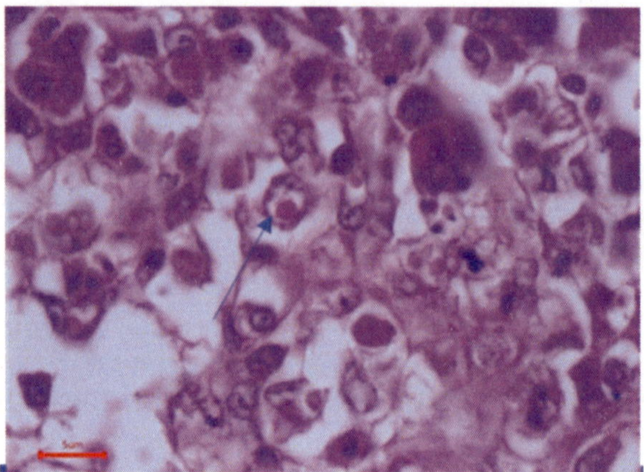

Inclusion Body Hepatitis-Chicken-Eosinophilic intranuclear inclusion bodies (Arrow)

Degenerations

1. Acute Cell Swelling

- This occurs whenever the cells are incapable of maintaining ionic and fluid homeostasis.
- It is the first change to all forms of injury to the cell.
- It is difficult to appreciate the change with light microscopy.
- The organ is swollen.

Causes

As discussed in the reversible cell injury

Grossly

Organs appears pallor, increase in turgor, increase in weight when involves allcells in the organ.

Microscopically

Enlargement of cells is mostly observed in liver, convoluted tubules of the kidney, or in skeletal and cardiac muscle. Cytoplasm stains slightly more eosinophilic and more granular than normal. It is discernible by compression of microvasculature of organs. e.g. hepatic sinusoids and capillary network in renal cortex.

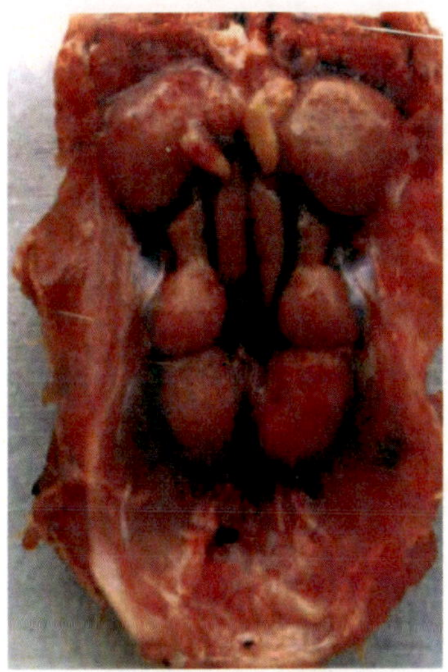

Chicken-Acute cell swelling - Swollen kidneys

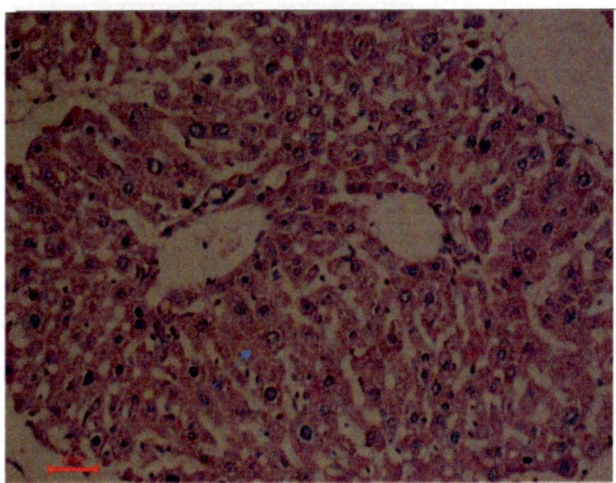

Liver-Cell swelling-Narrowing of sinusoid (Arrow)

2. Hydropic Degeneration

A variant of cell swelling with excessive accumulation of fluid leading to even bursting of cells. It is caused by more severe irritant.

Causes

Physical causes

- Rubbing
- Friction injury

- Axe handling
- Ill fitting shoes, saddle

Thermal injuries

- Fire accident
- Hot substances – water and oil
- Blisters are seen.

Chemicals

- Application of croton oil, red iodide of mercury

Infectious agents

- FMD in cattle – vesicles
- Pox – blisters in stratified squamous epithelium

Neoplasm

- Cervical cancer

Grossly

- Blisters are seen on skin.
- Fluid escapes on incision and blister collapses consequently.

Microscopically

- Cells are swollen.
- Cytoplasm shows vacuoles which represent distended and sequestrated segments of endoplasmic reticulum. Cells may enlarge with coalition of fluid and may burst showing blisters and vesicles.
- Skin-Prickle cell layer is affected.
- Eosin stains cytoplasm pink depending on protein content. Using negative method of staining i.e. staining of fat or glycogen, vacuoles with water are identified.

Sequelae

- Healing occurs rapidly in uncomplicated cases without scar formation.
- Invasion of pyogenic bacteria like streptococci and staphylococci may cause abscesses or septicaemia.

3. Mucinous or Mucous Degeneration

- Mucinous or mucous degeneration is the excessive accumulation of mucin in degenerating epithelium cell.
- Mucin is **glassy, viscid, stringy, slimy glycoprotein** normally produced by epithelium cell lining mucous membranes.
- **Mucus** is mucin mixed with water.

Causes

- It is caused by mild irritant.
- Mechanical or chemical injury (Disinfectant or soap).
- Thermal injury by heat or cold
- Infectious diseases – Canine distemper, bovine viral diarrhoea

Grossly

- Mucous covering is seen as clear transparent material on mucous membrane which is stringy and slimy inconsistency. e.g. common cold.
- Mucosa is hyperaemic.
- In estrus, large amount of mucous is normally produced which may be hanging from vulva of cattle.

Microscopically

- Cytoplasm shows small droplets of mucous which may coalesce forming large droplets displacing nucleus to side and compressing the nuclei.
- As the mucin accumulation continues the cell ruptures and desquamated.
- Haematoxylin stains the mucin blue.
- Mucicarmine and PAS stains the mucin red.

Sequelae

- On removal of the causative agent, epithelium lost is repaired by regeneration following stoppage of overproduction of mucin.

4. Mucoid or Myxomatous Degeneration

- Mucoid (Resemble mucin/mucin - like) is a glycoprotein similar to mucin in connective tissue found in foetus but not in adult tissue.

Causes

- Neoplasm of connective tissue e.g. Myxoma and myxosarcoma
- Thyroid deficiency in human –myxoedema
- Cachexia, starvation, parasitism or chronic disease

Grossly

- Adipose tissue shows the change. Affected tissue is shrunken, flabby, flaccid in consistency and has translucent jelly-like appearance.

Microscopically

- Degenerated tissue stains intensely blue with haematoxylin, nuclei are hyperchromatic and intercellular fluid takes slight bluish tinge.

Sequelae

- In cachexia, the fat becomes normal on correction of condition.
- Tumours indicate embryonal nature and it is unfavourable.
- Pseudomucin which resembles mucin is secreted by ovarian cystadenomas and parovarian cysts.
- Pseudomucin is not precipitated by acetic acid and stains pink with eosin whereas mucin is precipitated by acetic acid and stains blue with haematoxylin. Pseudomucin is not harmful and secretion of a normal cell.

5. Hyaline Degeneration (Hyaline Change)

(**L. hyaline** – **glassy**) It is the descriptive terminology of microscopical appearance.

Affected tissue appears homogenous glassy and pink in H & E staining. It may be found in different conditions.

- Keratohyaline
- Cellular hyaline
- Connective tissue hyaline
- Keratohyaline

It is normally found in stratum corneum.

Pathological amounts of keratohyaline

- Mechanical injury - e.g. saddles and harness
- Papillomas in dogs and cats
- Chlorinated naphthalene poisoning in cattle causes hyperkeratosis
- Hypovitaminosis A –keratinization of epithelium of digestive and upper respiratory tract
- May be protective but the condition like corns may be very painful. Removal of the cause results in desquamation of excessive keratohyaline and epithelium becomes normal.

a. Cellular Hyaline

- The dead cells are kneaded together forming homogenous mass resembling sand; since it stains with iodine it is called **corpora amylacea** (**Starch-like**).

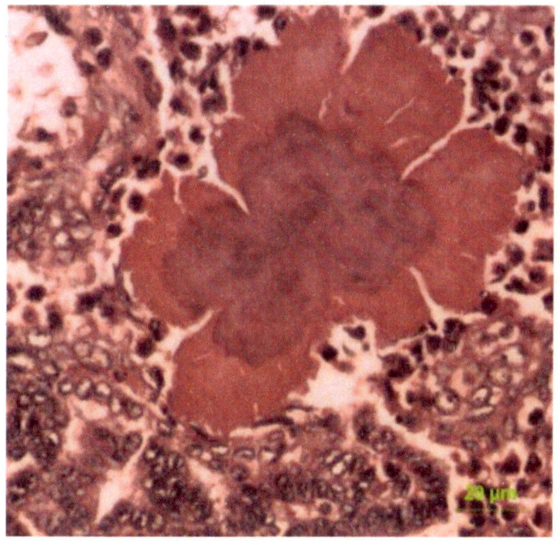

Corpora amylacea- Dog-Mammary Tumour

- They are commonly seen in prostate.
- They are observed in lungs in pneumonia, pulmonary infarction, mammary glands of cows which are dried off quickly, in brain as **brain sand**, in islets of Langerhans in diabetes and in renal nephritis as the renal tubular epithelium gets desquamated and forms hyaline cast with albumin.

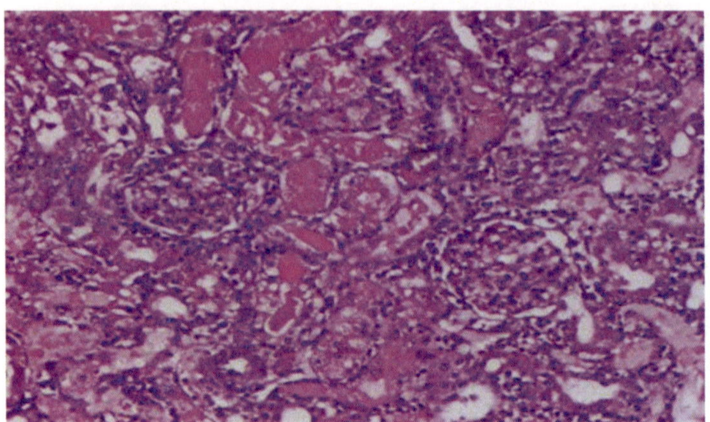

Hyaline cast with tubular epithelial cell degeneration and necrosis-Dog-Kidney

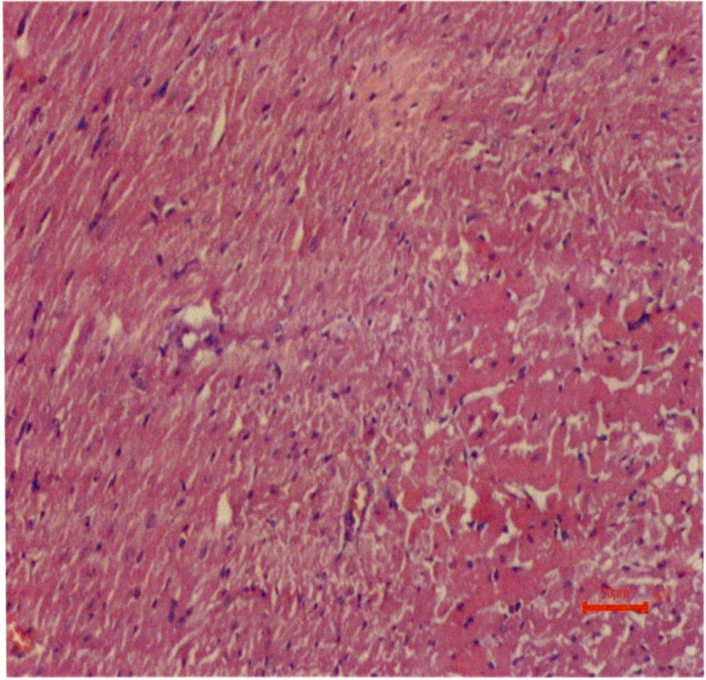

Hyaline degeneration of myocytes- Heart-Dog

b. Connective Tissue Hyaline

- This is found in old scars, degenerating stroma of tumours, lymph nodes in chronic inflammation and arteriosclerosis.
- This is permanent change persisting for life.

Gout

- The gout is defined as increase in the amount of deposition of uric acid and urates in tissue (viscera and joints).
- This is mainly observed in birds in which the end product of protein metabolism is uric acid (insoluble in water) and is produced in liver. Mammals are ureotelic organisms i.e. urea is the end product of protein metabolism which is water soluble.

There are two types of gouts

- Visceral gout
- Articular gout

Causes

It is mainly due to

- Failure of urinary excretion of urates
- Obstruction of ureters
- Renal damage
- Dehydration (common with water deprivation)
- Hypovitaminosis A
- Oosporin (mycotoxicosis)
- Sodium bicarbonate treatment
- Hyperuricaemia is the result in sodium bicarbonate toxicity.
- It is the sequel of alkalosis with protein breakdown.
- It is found only at necropsy.

Visceral gout

- The deposits of urates are found in kidney, serous surfaces of heart, mesentery, air sacs and peritoneum and in severe cases deposition are found in the synovial sheath, tendons, joints and muscular surfaces.
- It appears as white chalky coat.

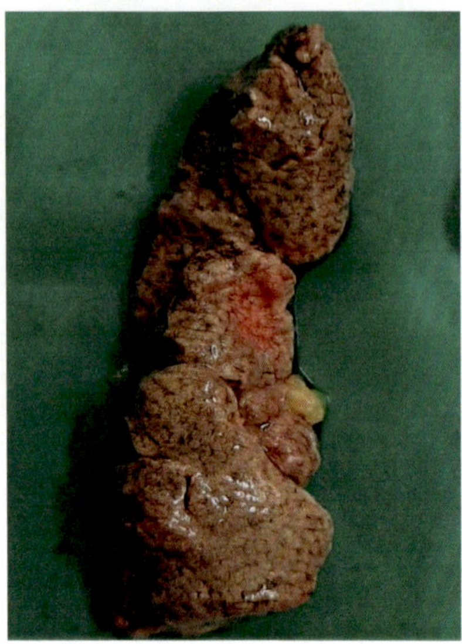

Visceral Gout-Kidney-Chicken- Urate deposits

Microscopically

- Urate crystals found in clusters which are pale elongated and needle shaped.
- It is surrounded by inflammatory cells like heterophils, lymphocytes and foreign body giant cells and fibroblasts.
- On H & E section, it appears as clefts.
- Gout-Kidney- Urate deposits
- It is a sporadic problem.

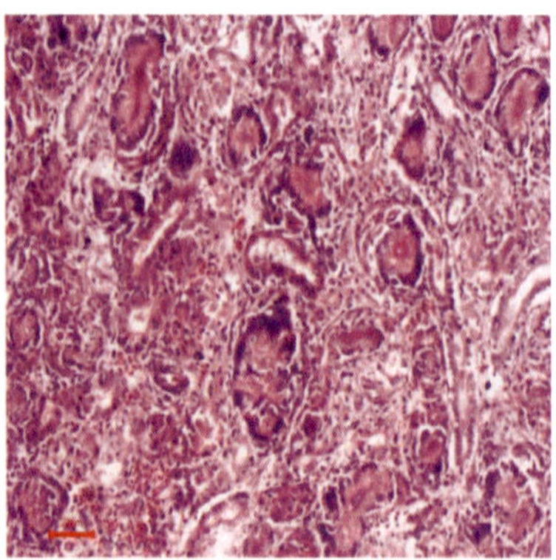

Visceral Gout-Kidney- Urate deposits and giant cells Articular gout

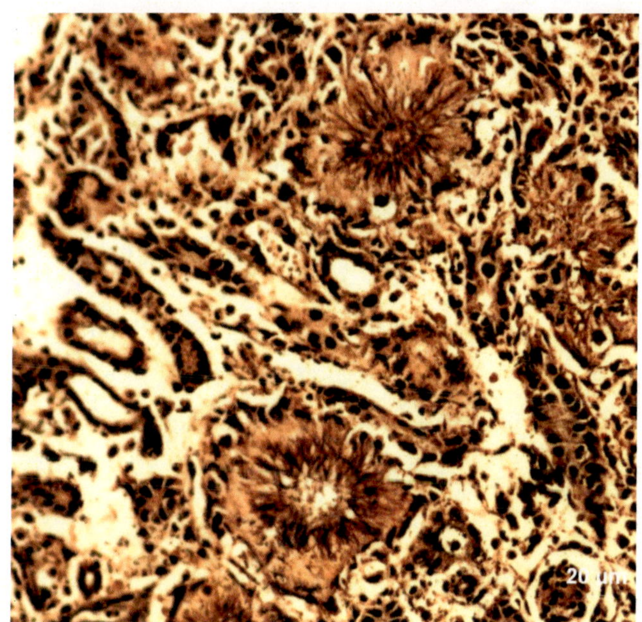

Visceral Gout-DeGalantha stain-Black coloured needle shaped urate crystals

Clinical signs

- Leg shifting, lameness and inability to bend the toes are observed.
- Tophi are characteristics of articular gout which are deposition of urates around joints particularly of the feet.
- The joints are enlarged with deformed feet.
- Deposits are seen as white semifluid substance.

Necrosis

Necrosis (Gr. Nekrosis-Deadness) is defined as local death of cells in a tissue in a living animal.

Grossly

Necrotic tissue is pale, grayish white, dull and depressed surrounded by hyperaemic zone.

Microscopically

Nuclear changes are characteristic. These are

- **Pyknosis (Gr.Pykno-Thick,dense):** Shrinkage or condensation of nucleus which takes up deep blue colour. The chromatin condenses to a structureless mass.
- **Karyorrhexis** (Gr. Karyo-Nucleus; rhexis-Fragmentation): Fragmentation of nucleus
- **Karyolysis** (Gr. Karyo-Nucleus; Lysis-Dissolution): Dissolution or disappearance of nucleus
- Cytoplasm is swollen, homogeneous and stained intensely pink due to decreased basophilia with loss of ribosomes.

Types of necrosis

Depending on the gross and microscopic features necrosis is divided into following four types

1. Coagulative necrosis
2. Caseation necrosis
3. Liquefactive/suppurative necrosis
4. Fat necrosis

1. Coagulative Necrosis

"While architectural details of tissue are retained, the structural details are lost due to necrosis"

- This type of necrosis occurs due to ischaemia, white muscle disease in vitamin E and selenium deficiency, necrosis of liver in *Fusobacterium sphaerophorus* infection, mercuric toxicity in renal tubular epithelial cells and cutaneous or mucosal epithelium in contact poison with phenol.
- **Grossly,** the necrotic tissue is dry, white or grayish white and homogeneous and slightly depressed from the surrounding healthy tissue.

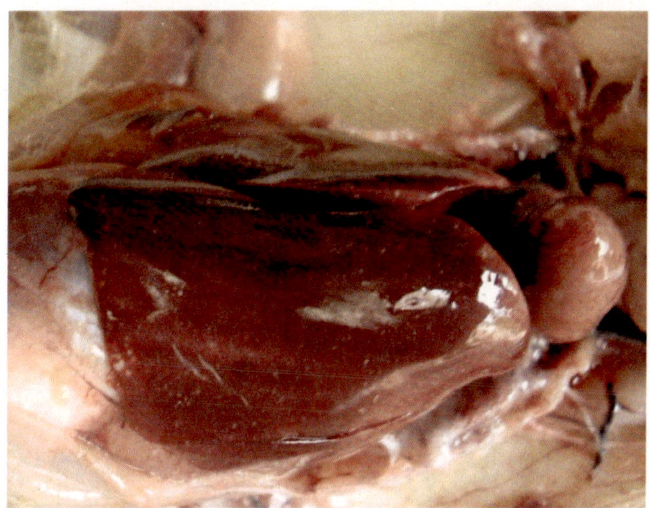

Chicken-Fowl Cholera-Liver-Multifocal military necrosis

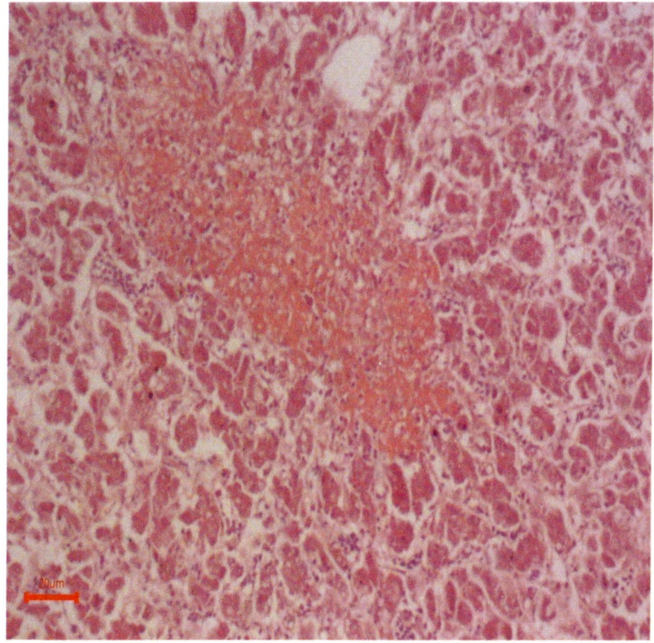

Chicken-Fowl Cholera-Liver-Hepatocellular coagulative necrosis

Microscopically, the architectural details of the area are maintained and cellular details are lost.

• This is due to blockage of proteolysis with denaturation of proteins including enzymatic proteins of the cell.

- The cellular shape is preserved and nuclear details are lost (Nuclei show pyknosis, karyorrhexis and karyolysis or absence).
- The cytoplasm appears homogeneous and eosinophilic due to coagulation of protein. It takes long time for the removal of dead materials because the autolytic enzymes are destroyed and no leukocytic responses.
- This type of necrosis is characteristically found in parenchymatous organs like kidney, liver and muscle except the brain.

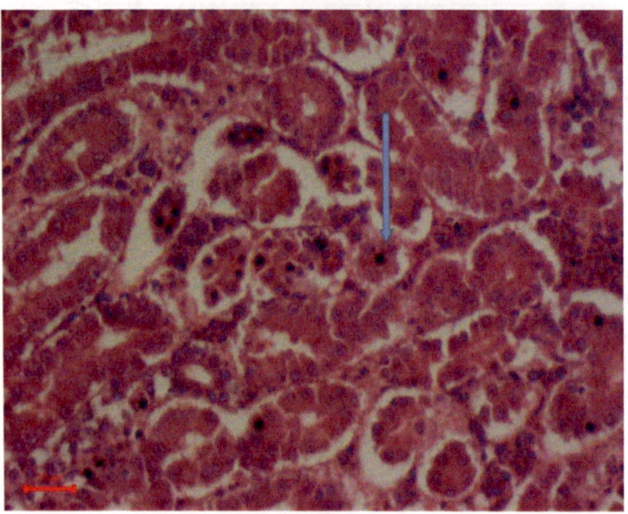

Kidney-Tubular epithelial cell- Pyknosis (Condensation of nucleus) (Blue arrow)

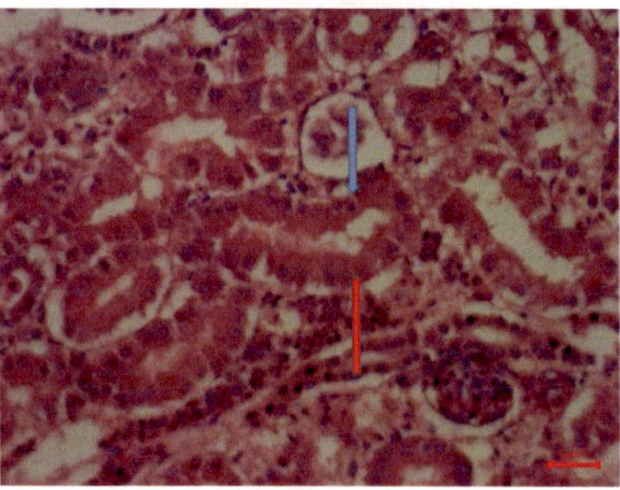

Kidney-Tubular epithelial cell-Pyknosis (Blue arrow); Karyolysis (Red arrow)

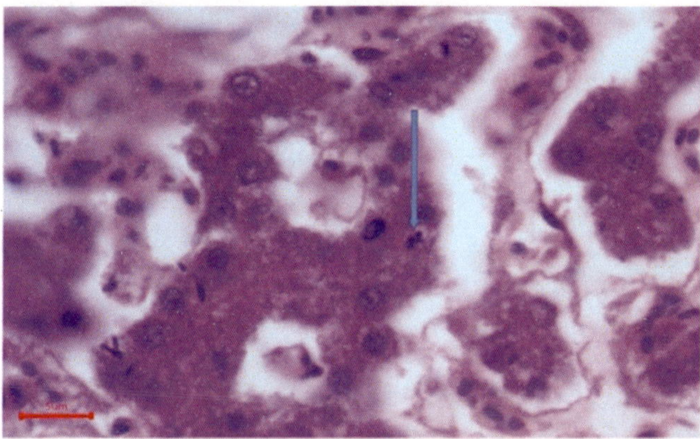

Kidney-Tubular epithelial cell-Karyolysis (Blue arrow)

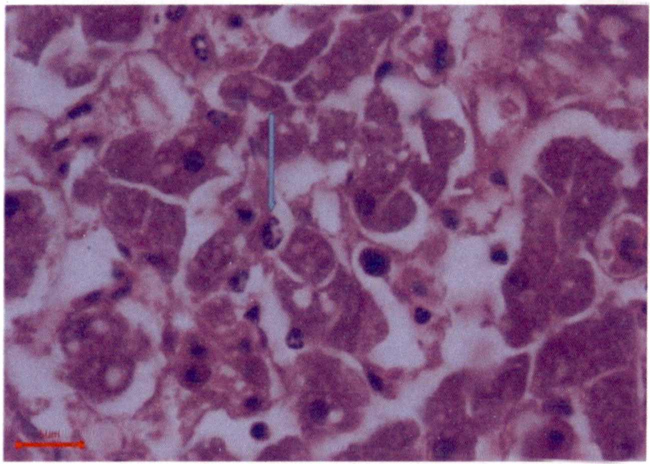

Kidney-Tuber epithelial cell-Chromatin margination (Blue arrow)

2. Caseous Necrosis (L. Caseous-Cheese)

- The architectural and cellular details are lost. This is more chronic type of lesion often associated with poorly degraded lipid materials of bacterial origin. This type of necrosis occurs in *Mycobacterium tuberculosis* infection, oesophagostomosis and caseous lymphadenitis in sheep and tularaemia in primates.
- **Grossly**, the necrotic tissue is converted into a homogeneous, soft, friable, grayish white cheesy granular mass. The dead tissue attracts calcium deposits and is enclosed within a connective tissue capsule.

- **Microscopically**, structure less, amorphous necrotic area surrounded by epithelioid cells, giant cells, lymphocytes and plasma cells with central area of dystrophic calcification

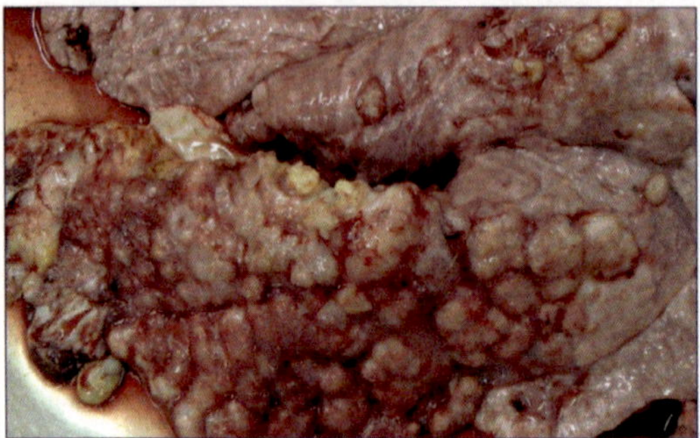

Caseation Necrosis- Nodular lesions-Tuberculosis-Lung

3. Liquefactive Necrosis

- **Necrotic tissue is liquid in consistency**. It is especially seen in the central nervous system (malacia) and any infection with pyogenic bacteria leading to pus formation (Abscess).
- The former is due to severe hypoxic or toxic injury with focal dissolution of the neuropil.
- The later is due to autolysis or heterolysis from enzymes of neutrophils leading to collection of pus containing necrotic tissue, microorganisms and dead neutrophils (Suppuration).
- Liquefactive necrosis - Pyometra
- The pus becomes caseous and insipid if stands for longer time.

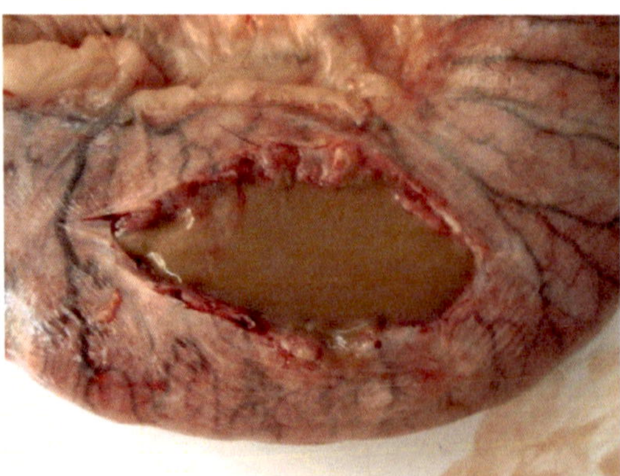

Pyometra- Note the presence of pus in the uterus of a bitch

- **Microscopically,** the pus or the purulent area shows dark, contracted and agranular neutrophils with varying amounts of tissue debris, fibrin and plasma proteins.
- **An abscess is a localized collection of pus (Liquefactive necrosis)** caused by suppuration, deep in tissues.
- The process is designed to contain the pathogenic organisms and sequestering necrotic tissue from spreading in the animal.
- The pyogenic organisms cause localized necrosis and attract neutrophils to the necrotic spaces.
- This is a part of inflammatory response.

4. Fat Necrosis

It is death of adipose tissue in a living animal. Three types of fat necrosis are described

i. Enzymatic fat necrosis

ii. Traumatic fat necrosis

iii. Nutritional fat necrosis

i. Enzymatic fat necrosis

- It is commonly found in steatitis (Inflammation of fat) and other inflammatory lesions affecting adipose tissue e.g. Pancreatic fat

Pathogenesis

- In acute pancreatic necrosis and pancreatitis, the lipase released from acinar cells gets activated and saponification occurs by digestion of triglycerides into glycerol and fatty acids.
- Glycerol being water soluble, is absorbed. The released fatty acids when combine with calcium results in the presence of chalky white flakes.

Grossly, hard, white, opaque masses resembling that of soap flakes are seen. The fat loses yellow translucent nature.

Microscopically, necrotic adipocytes may show eosinophilic shadow outlines, become basophilic due to dystrophic calcification and surrounded by inflammatory reactions along the area due to acute to chronic injury.

- Fat solvents do not remove necrotic fat.

ii. Traumatic fat necrosis

- It results from mechanical injury to adipose tissue.
- **Causes**: working, biting, parturition (perivaginal fat in cattle, subcutaneous and intramuscular fat in recumbent cattle)
- **Grossly**, firm, opaque, chalky masses found in the area with acute to chronic inflammatory reaction.
- **Example:** Abdominal fat necrosis in cattle
- Mesenteric, omental and retroperitoneal fat show necrosis containing large masses. Stenosis of intestine may occur in extreme cases.

iii. Nutritional fat necrosis

- This is the result of necrotic alteration in fat associated with extreme emaciation. e.g. Tuberculosis and Johne's disease in cattle and sheep.
- Grossly, necrotic fat is opaque, foamy and chalky white and may be calcified.
- Microscopically, necrotic adipocytes are pale pink (eosinophilic) and show numerous clubs (fatty acids) and crystals.
- The derivatives of fat, glycerol dissolves in body fluids, and fatty acid crystals dissolve in fat solvents leaving clefts.
- Calcified area is basophilic, surrounded by chronic inflammatory reaction.
- Differential diagnosis: Inflammatory reaction and calcification are lacking in autolytic fat.

Apoptosis

Apoptosis is programmed cell death in which there is death of individual cells in death processes.

In embryogenesis and normal growth, physiologic cell death occurs which may be referred as programmed cell death. Apoptosis can also occur in pathologic diseases.

Mechanism of Apoptosis

There are two processes

1. Initiation phase mediated by caspases
2. Execution phase in which enzymatic degradation leads to cell death

1. Initiation Phase

There are two pathways of initiation of apoptosis.

i. Extrinsic receptor initiated pathway

ii. Intrinsic mitochondrial pathway

These two pathways are interconnected and converge to activate caspases

Extrinsic pathway

- On cross linkage of Fas (Death domain) by its ligand three or molecules come together and bind to cytoplasmic Fas-associated death domain (FADD) which in turn binds to inactive forms of caspase-8 via death domain.
- These activated caspases trigger a cascade of caspase activation and mediate execution phase of apoptosis. FLIP protein inhibits apoptosis by binding to procaspase-8.
- This mechanism is used to protect infected normal cells from Fas mediated apoptosis.

Intrinsic mitochondrial pathway

- There are more than 20 antiapoptotic proteins. Of which Bcl-2 and Bcl-x are located on the mitochondrial membrane of cytoplasm. Bcl-2 and Bcl-x are replaced when cells are deprived of survival signals or stress by proapoptotic members like Bak, Bax and Bim.
- This leads to increased mitochondrial membrane permeability and release of several proteins which activate caspase cascade e.g. cytochrome C from mitochondria which binds to Apaf-1(Apoptosis activating factor-1protein).

The complex activates caspase-9.Apoptosis activating factor from mitochondria also neutralizes various apoptotic inhibitors which block caspase activation

2. Execution Phase

- The final proteolytic cascade is mediated by the proteases (Caspase: 'c'-cystine protease that cleaves aspartic acid residues).
- There are more than 10 members in caspase family which are grouped into initiator and executioner groups depending on their order in which they are activated during apoptosis e.g. caspase-8 and 9 are initiator caspases and caspase-3 and 6 are executioner caspases.

- These caspases are hydrolysed autocatalytically following cleavage of initiator caspase to generate the active form.
- The enzymatic death programme sets in motion by rapid and sequential activation of other caspases.
- These caspases can act on many cellular components like cytoskeleton and nuclear matrix proteins.
- Cytoskeleton destruction and nuclear break down occurs.
- Caspase target proteins of transcription, DNA replication and DNA repair in the nucleus e.g. caspase-3 activates cytoplasmic DNAs.

Not only gross changes, but microscopical changes are also not obvious since single cell death occurs.

Microscopically

i. **Cell shrinkage:** In the individual cells: cells-size smaller, cytoplasm is dense and organelles are tightly packed.

ii. **Condensation of chromatins: Most characteristic in apoptosis.** Aggregation of chromatins under nuclear membrane with variable shape and size (Semilunar shape)

iii. **Cytoplasmic fragmentation**

iv. **Cytoplasmic buds containing fragments of nucleus:** Cytoplasm shows excessive surface budding and formation of membrane bound fragments (Apoptotic bodies) containing cytoplasm and tightly packed organelles with or without nuclear fragments. Nucleus itself may break up into two or more fragments

v. **Presence of apoptotic bodies in the adjacent cells and phagocytes**

vi. **Inflammation is absent.**

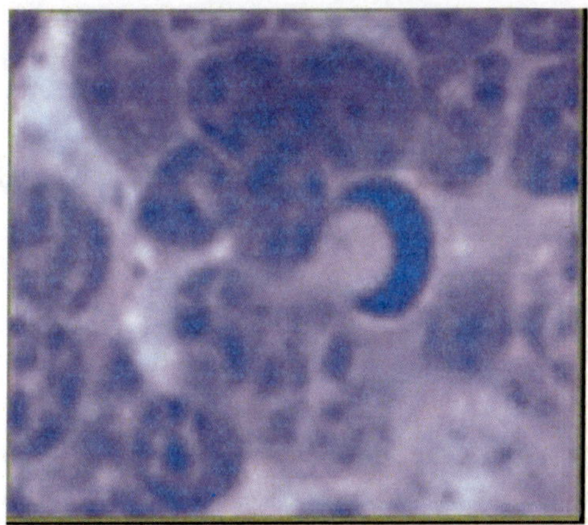

Apoptotic cell-Lymphocyte-Nucleus-Note crescent shaped chromatin margination

Post Mortem Autolysis and Necrosis

Difference between post mortem autolysis and necrosis

S.No.	Post mortem autolysis	Necrosis
1.	Absence of inflammatory reaction	Presence of inflammatory reaction
2.	Autolytic changes are seen uniform throughout the tissue	Diffuse or focal adjacent living and dead tissues are seen.

Post-Mortem (PM) Changes

Somatic Death

- Somatic death is the death of the body as a whole.
- When respiration and cardiac action have stopped, the animal is said to have undergone somatic death.
- After death, the cells undergo certain changes (post mortem changes), which a pathologist must have knowledge of to distinguish them from lesions found in disease.

By a careful study of a postmortem changes one can determine the probable time of death and this is of great importance in veterolegal cases.

Factors influencing the Rate of Postmortem Autolysis

Species of animal: Pig-soft and moist muscle- rapid in onset, Horse-dry and firm muscle-slow in onset

Organ involved: The degrees of the expression of postmortem changes vary from tissue to tissue. The presence of bacterial flora, enzyme secretions and the availability of moisture and substrates influence the rate of postmortem autolysis. Pancreas-high amount of enzymes-rapid changes. Fibrous tissue-less amount of enzymes-slow changes. Retina-most sensitive, separates from choroids. Adrenals, liver, testis and abdominal organs also show early autolytic changes.

Putrefaction (Decomposition)

- Decomposition of tissues brought about by the protein splitting anaerobic saprophytic organisms, results in the formation of gas and variety of foul smelling substances- ammonia, hydrogen sulphide, indol, skatol and putrescent amines-like “putriscience and cadaverine”.
- The tissue turns black or dark-green as a result of formation of iron sulphide from break down of haemoglobin.
- The common putrefactive organisms involved are *Clostridium spp* normally present in faeces, that cause pronounced postmortem changes in the body like gaseous distension, softening etc.
- Bacterial flora present in GIT and respiratory tract bring about the post-mortem changes rapidly under favourable conditions

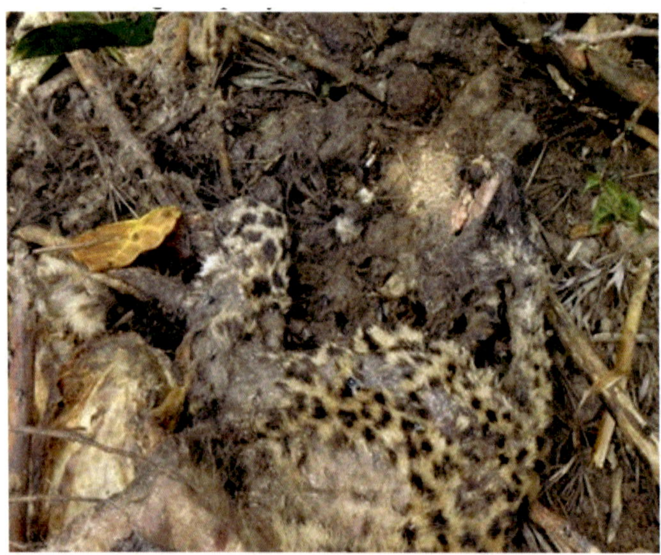

Leopard-PM decomposition

Sequence of Postmortem Changes

- Algor mortis
- Rigor mortis
- Livor mortis- hypostatic congestion
- PM clotting of blood
- Imbibition of hemoglobin
- Imbibition of bile
- PM desquamation
- PM softening
- PM discoloration
- PM distention
- PM displacement
- PM rupture of organ and tissue

1. Algor Mortis

Algor mortis is cooling of the body. It commences at or before the stoppage of blood flow. The rate of cooling depends on the following factors:

- External atmospheric temperature
- Air currents
- The thickness of hair coat or wool
- Adiposity of the animal
- Amount of fermentable ingesta in the digestive tract
- Larger animals cool slowly; so also in sheep, with thick wool cooling occurs slowly. Limbs and other extremities cool more rapidly than the trunk.

The rate at which post mortem changes takes place depends on the rate of cooling and other factors detailed below

A. Surrounding External Atmospheric Temperature

- Since the postmortem changes are brought about by enzymatic and bacterial activity, high temperature that accelerates this activity will naturally bring on the post mortem changes soon.

- So in summer, the carcass putrefies quickly. Cold on the other hand retards the enzymatic and bacterial activity.
- Freezing and deep freezing may stop the activity completely.
- Hence, carcasses are in perfect state of preservation under polar ice-caps for considerable length of time.

B. State of the Body at the time of Death

- Higher the temperature at death, sooner do postmortem changes commence

C. State of Muscular Activity of Animal Prior to Death

- In animals, that have been very active prior to death post mortem changes commence quicker. This is found in animals that die in chase. Similarly, animals that are killed or die of strychnine poisoning and in animals that die of tetanus, postmortem changes appear early.
- The reasons are

  a) higher body temperature

  b) greater production of lactic acid in muscular contractions and exercise

D. Size of Animal

- Since body cools slower and so heat is retained longer in larger animals, postmortem changes appear quicker in those animals.

E. External Coverings

- Since thick hair or wool retard heat, dissipation, postmortem changes are seen sooner in thick haired or coated animals.
- Fatness of animals

Fat is a poor conductor of heat and so heat loss in fat carcasses is slow, with resultant speedier onset of postmortem changes.

• Infection of Animals

Widespread bacterial infection, especially septiceamic in character, at the time of death begins on postmortem changes

The following are the changes noticed after death

2. Rigor Mortis

- Rigor mortis is contraction of muscles after death.
- There is a contraction of muscles after death so that the joints become stiff and body is rigid.
- Rigor mortis develops first in those muscles that are very active. e.g heart, palpebral muscles, muscles of the head and neck.
- Gradually other muscles of the forelimbs, the trunk and the hind limbs, are affected in that order.
- It passes of also in this order, starting first in the head. Usually, rigor mortis appears in 1 to 8 hours after death and may disappear from 20-30 hours.

The following factors hasten the onset of rigor mortis

a) High atmospheric temperature

b) Active exercise- hunting, fighting, racing or struggling

Causes of Rigor Mortis

- The exact mechanism is not known.
- After death, there is a great overturn of high energy phosphate bonds in the muscle. Adenosine triphosphate (ATP) which breaks down is resynthesized by the energy derived from glycosis.
- So long as ATP is present, rigors do not occur. With the exhaustion of glycogen, all of ATP is degraded and rigor occurs, since in the absence of ATP relaxation of muscles cannot occur.
- For the relaxation of the muscles to occur, a considerable quantity of ATP must be absorbed to the muscle proteins.
- Hence, onset of rigor is delayed in well fed animals with large quantities of stored muscle glycogen.
- But in starved animals, rigor naturally commences earlier. Subsequently when there is no longer any energy necessary for keeping up the chemical activity in the muscle fibres, rigor passes off.
- Onset of rigor mortis is slow in cold weather and in emaciated and cachectic animals.

- In the later, it is due to the complete exhaustion of chemical systems producing energy.

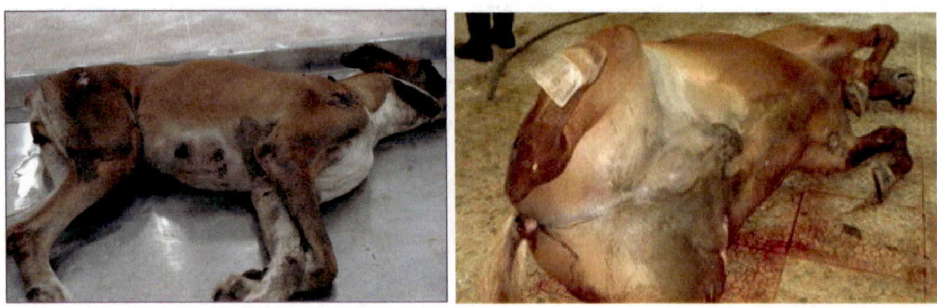

Rigor mortis-Dog-Absent Rigor mortis-Horse-Present

Livor mortis: **Hypostatic congestion** is, due to gravity, accumulation of blood in vessels of organs that are found on the lower side of the recumbent animal.

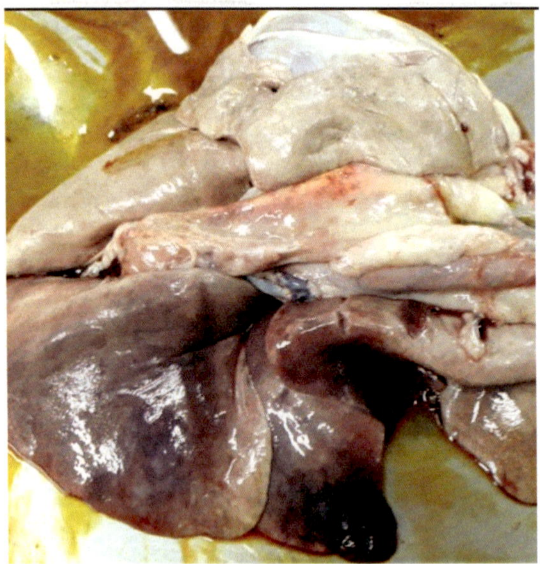

Sheep- Lung-Livor mortis-Hypostatic congestion

3. PM Clot: This is the coagulation of blood in the vessels after death. Chicken fat is the white clot while currant jelly clot is the red clot seen in the clot. PM clot is formed after death of animal.

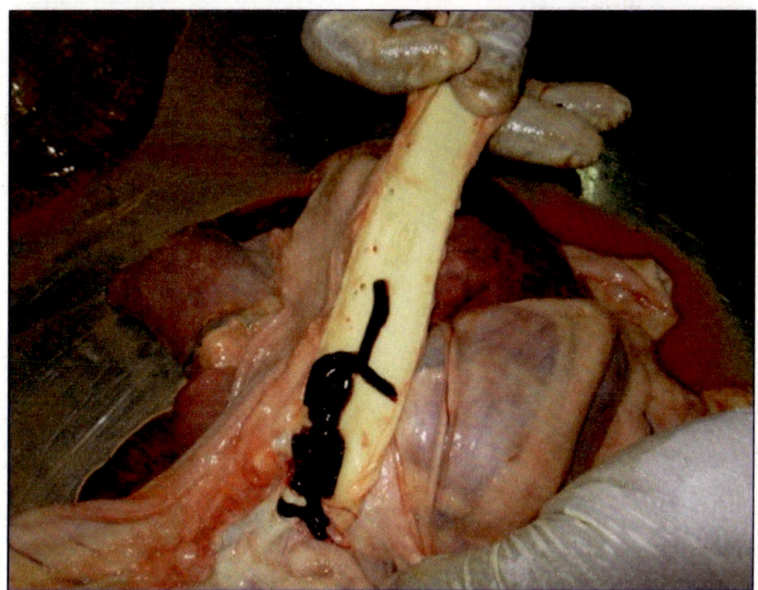

PM Clot- Smaller than vessel

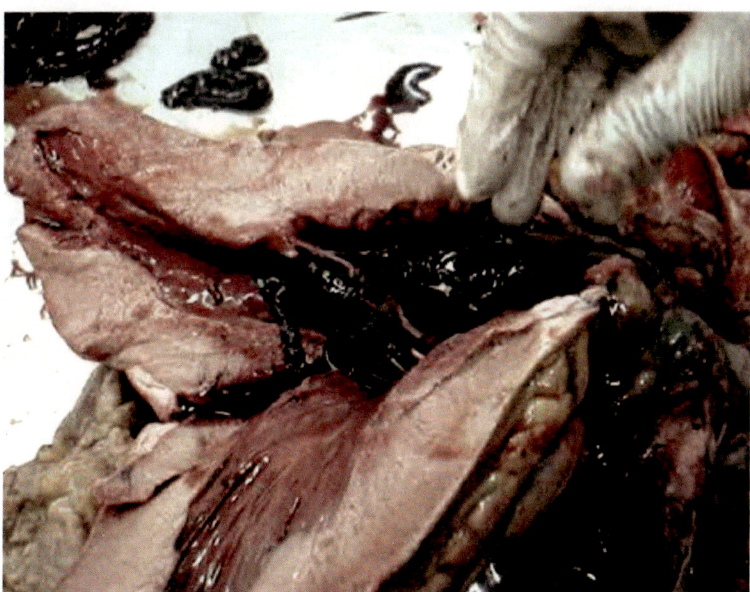

Cow-Heart-Post Mortem Clot; Haemoglobin imbibition is evident

4. Imbibition of Hemoglobin: PM staining is pinkish discolouration of endothelium of larger vessels due to haemoglobin (liberated from lysed erythrocytes) after death.

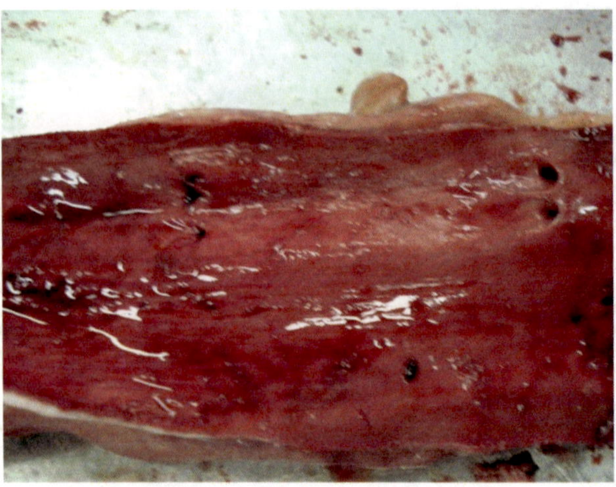

PM staining-Imbibition of haemoglobin-Cow-Aorta

5. PM imbibition of bile: This yellow pigmentation of the tissue occurring in the vicinity of gall bladder.

6. PM Softening: This is softening of tissues, after death, by the action of autolytic enzymes of the cells and the proteolytic ferments of the saprophytes and infecting bacteria.

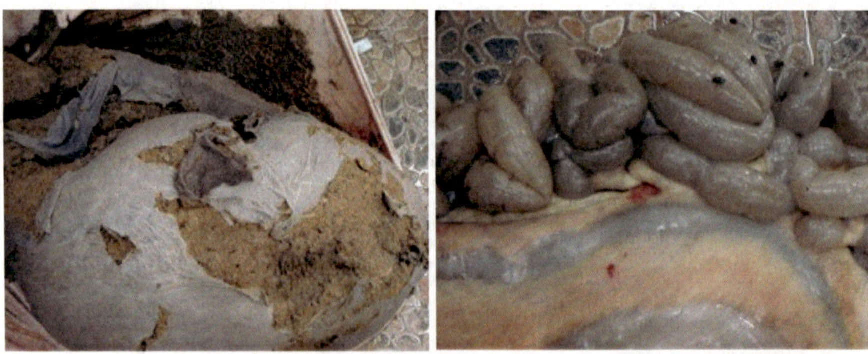

Cow-Rumen-Mucosa peeled off- Cow-PM softening; Intestine softening No inflammation

7. PM Discoloration: Pseudomelanosis coli is staining (blackish / greenish discolouration) of intestines due to formation of iron sulphide (H_2S + Fe from Hb = Iron sulphide) after death of animals.

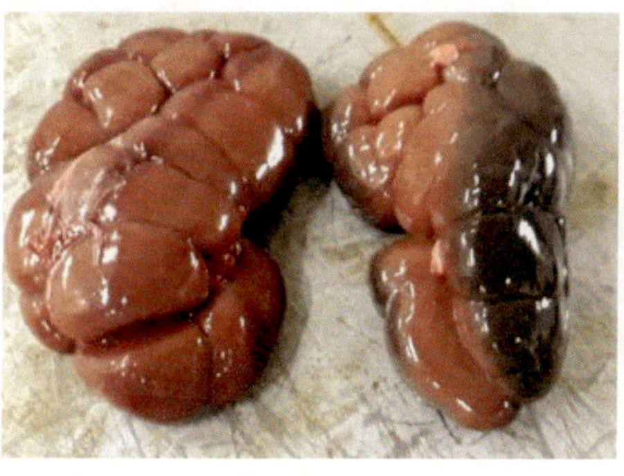

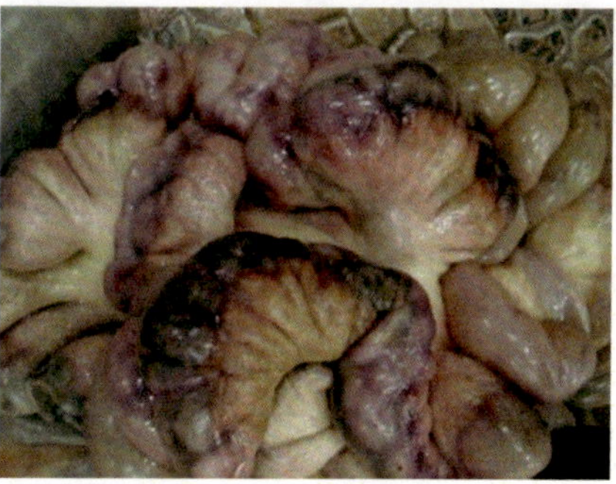

Cow-PM greenish discoloration-Kidney Cow- Pseudomelanosis coli-Intestine

8. PM bloat / PM emphysema: It is accumulation of gas in the rumen and intestines due to fermentation of food after death.

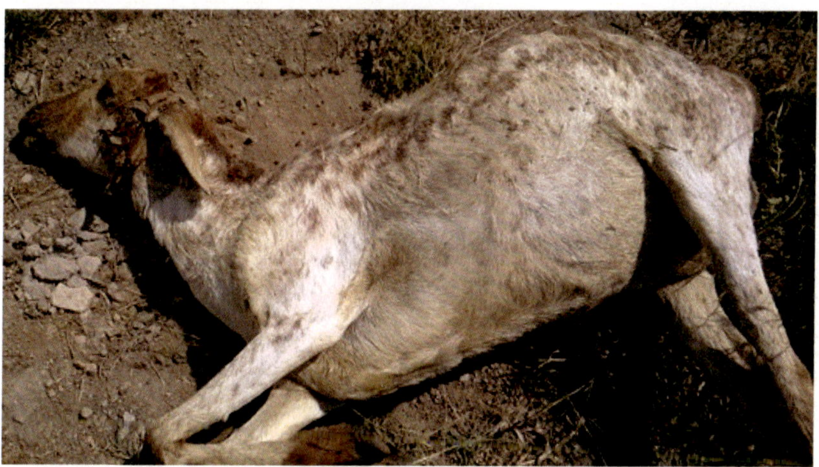

PM Bloat

9. PM displacement of Organs: This may occur following handling of carcass by rolling etc.

10. PM Rupture of Organ and Tissue: This may be attributed to softening and handling but devoid of any inflammatory reaction.

In equine practice, stud fee is payable only on the birth of a live foal.

So, the veterinarian may be required to certify as to whether a foal was born alive or dead.

The two criteria to be looked for are:

• Does the lung float in water?

If the lung floats the foal was born alive since presence of air renders the lung buoyant. If born dead, lung sinks in water.

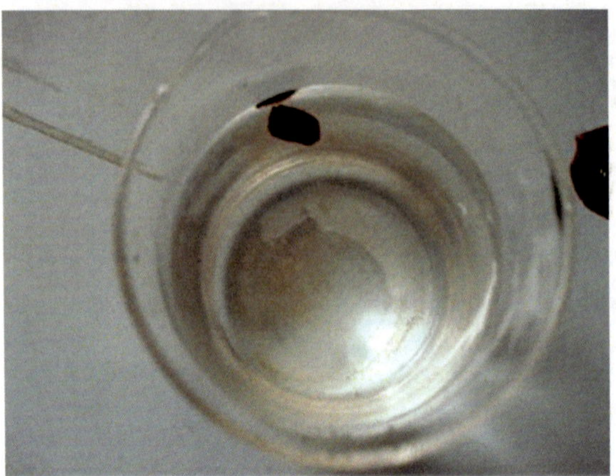

Bucket test- Lung Piece-Float-Live- In collapse or pneumonia, it will sink in water

Air can be present in lung only if the animal had breathed and breathing can occur only if the foal was born alive.

• Bucket test

Glass sealer-

Normal lung-Float in water

Collapsed/Pneumonic lung-Sink in water

• Did it suckle?

Presence of milk or curds in the stomach is valid evident that the foal was alive at birth and had suckled.

6

Gangrene

Definition

Gangrene is a necrotic area invaded by saprophytic organisms leading to putrefaction.

Types of Gangrene

There are three types of gangrene

1. Dry gangrene
2. Moist gangrene
3. Gas gangrene

1. Dry Gangrene

Dry gangrene represents an area of coagulation necrosis resulting from infarction followed by mummification. The extremities of the body like tail, ears, legs and udder are affected.

Causes

- **Toxins (phytotoxins and ergotoxins):** The toxins cause marked peripheral arteriolar vasoconstriction and damage to capillaries leading to thrombosis and infarction.
- Fescue poisoning
- **Cold (Frost bite):** Direct freezing and ice crystal formation leading to cellular damage, vascular damage and ischaemic necrosis.

Gross Pathology

- Affected part is dry (dehydration due to exposure to environment), shrivel (dehydration) and brown to black (due to formation of iron sulphide: iron from haemoglobin degradation, sulphide from putrefaction), proliferation of bacteria due to unfavourable environment, temperature and moisture.

- However, at the junction of living and dead tissue, there is a **line of demarcation** due to active inflammatory reaction.

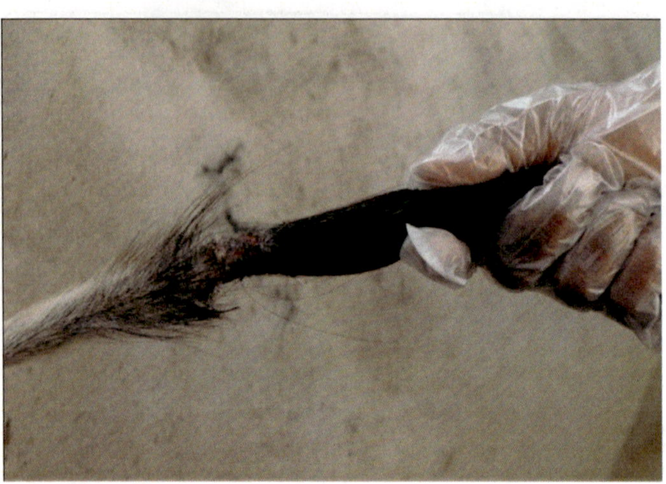

Dry Gangrene -Tail-Cow

2. Moist Gangrene

Causes: Displacements, Intussusception, volvulus, incarceration

Gross Pathology

- The affected parts are soft, moist and reddish brown to black, foul smelling or putrid odour due to hydrogen sulphide, ammonia and mercaptanes.
- The environment is conducive for rapid growth of bacteria. There is **no line of demarcation** between live and dead tissue.

Histopathology

- Initial coagulation necrosis with a few bacterial multiplications.
- Later liquified due to rapid proliferation of bacteria and infiltrating neutrophils

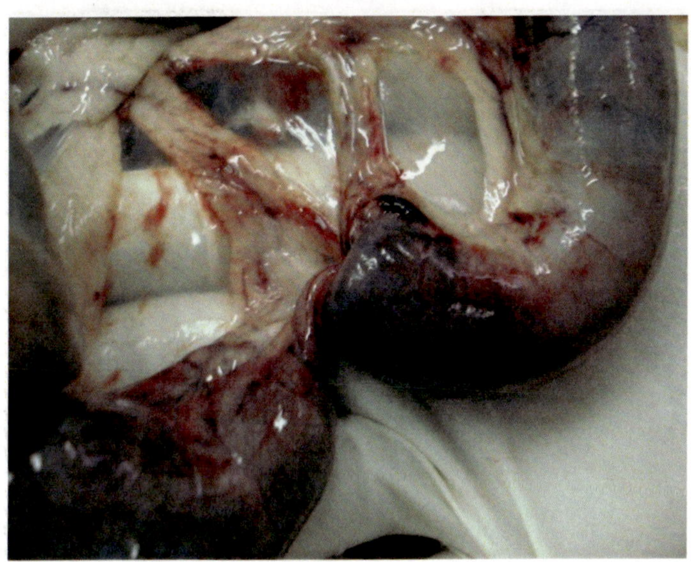

Moist Gangrene-Intussusception-Dog

Gas Gangrene

- Anaerobic bacterial proliferation producing toxin and damaging the tissues. These organisms produce gas.
- **Examples:** *Clostridium perfringens and Clostridium septicum* are introduced by penetrating wounds.
- The clostridia proliferate in necrotic tissue under anaerobic environment and produce toxin which cause tissue damage.
- The *Clostridia chauvoei* spreads haematogenously from the intestine and lodge in muscle which requires some injury and necrosis for the spores to germinate and bacteria to proliferate.

Gross Pathology

Affected parts are dark red to black, contain gas bubbles, serosanguineous exudates and foul smelling.

Histopathology

Coagulative necrosis of muscle, bacteria, serosanguineous exudates and gas bubbles are seen.

7

Major Exogenous and Endogenous Pigments

Colouring Agents

Colouring agents are called as pigments. Tissues may be discoloured (e.g. Jaundice, tattoo) or excessively coloured (e.g. Melanosis) in diseases.

Origin

- External or exogenous pigments
- Internal or endogenous pigments

Exogenous Pigmentations

In exogenous pigmentations colouring substances can enter the body by three different routes.

- Respiratory route by inhalation
- Alimentary route by ingestion
- Cutaneous route by injection

Of these three entries, entry through respiratory route is the most common pathway for exogenous pigmentations.

- This results in pneumoconiosis characterized by pigmentation and fibrosis.
- **Pneumoconiosis** is a general term applied for any permanent deposition of substantial amounts of particulate matter in lung disease by inhalation;

Exogenous Pigmentations

Depending upon the type of exogenous pigment, the conditions are termed as follows

- Coal dust-Anthracosis
- Stone dust -Silicosis
- Iron dust -Siderosis
- Cotton dust -Byssinosis
- Asbestos dust-Asbestosis
- Fine stone dust or cement-Chalicosis
- Tin oxide-Stannosis
- Barium oxide-Baritosis

Anthracosis

Anthracosis is deposition of carbon particles in the lungs.

Sources: Air pollution (Near busy high ways industrial areas, coal mines- zoo animals and dogs)

Coal mines (Horses and mules -Olden days used to carry coal)

- The carbon particles inhaled are phagocytized by alveolar macrophages and transported through regional tracheobronchial lymph nodes.
- Carbon particles could not be digested.
- The carbon particle being inert is not metabolized by the body and hence remains in the tissue permanently.

Grossly

- The lung shows peppered appearance.
- The carbon deposits in sub-pleural area are seen as black foci.
- Regional lymph nodes may show carbon deposits in the medulla because of concentration of sinus macrophages in that location.
- Mild irritant, large scale fibrosis not seen. If combined with silicosis, fibrosis occurs. e.g. mine workers

Microscopically

- Fine black granules may be found within the macrophages or deposited extracellularly in the lungs (alveolar wall) or around the peribronchial areas.

- The pigments are resistant to solvents of bleaching agents and non-reactive.
- The carbon being mildly irritant elicits slight pulmonary fibrosis.

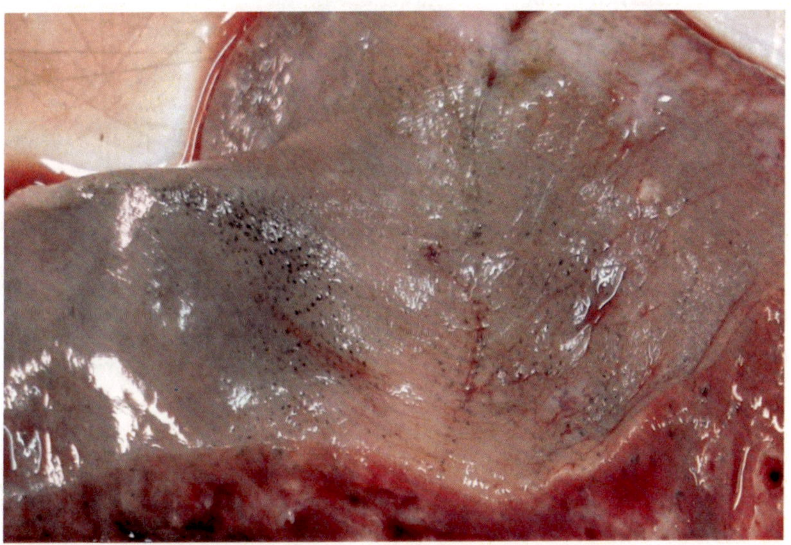

Note black carbon particle deposits

- Heavy deposits of carbon particles seen in human or animals living in highly polluted areas or occupational hazard-mine workers, ponies, horses. "Miner's lung in human.

Anthracosis-Lung

Silicosis

Silicosis is deposition of silicon in the lung.

- The condition is more common in human beings than in animals as an occupational hazard who are working in mines and quarries.
- Silicon; Silicon dioxide , amorphous or crystalline
- The crystalline form of silicon is more harmful irritant than amorphous form.
- The silicon is a powerful irritant and is insoluble in body fluids.

Gross Pathology: Lung shows multiple, small discrete nodules in the parenchyma.

- Similar lesions may also be found in the regional lymph nodes and pleura.
- Extensive fibrosis may predispose to pulmonary tuberculosis. **Microscopically,** the nodular regions are replaced by concentric layers of hyalinized collagen.

Tattoo

- Tattooing is a method of identification of animals in which the carbon pigments used are deposited in the dermis.
- Coloring pigments: Prussian blur reaction, Indian Ink, mercuric sulphide(vermillon), china ink, Bismark brown etc.
- Generally no harm
- The carbon pigments may be found as phagocytosed by macrophages or remains free in tissue.
- It evokes no inflammatory reaction.

Carotenoid pigments

Lipochrome pigments, not lipofuscin pigments.

Sources: β-carotene and fat soluble phyto-pigments

Grossly

- The pigments are normally found in the cells like adrenal cortex, corpus luteum, Kupffer and testicular cells and in plasma/serum and fat of horses and Jersey cattle.
- The fat is discoloured to yellow to orange-yellow. Holstein cattle, sheep, goat and cats store little or no carotenoids in which fat is white and serum is clear.
- In starvation fat atrophy, the adipocytes become dark yellowish brown due to concentration of carotenoids.

Microscopically

- Pigments are not seen due to dissolution of pigments by alcohol and clearing agents (Fat soluble nature).

Tetracyclines

Deciduous teeth or developing teeth and bone may show yellow or brown deposits if the animals are treated with tetracycline antibiotics.

Plumbism

Plumbism is deposition of lead in the body in chronic poisoning.

Sources : Ingestion of lead containing grains, paint, water, fodder, lead containing batteries, pastures containing lead ore etc.

- Lead water pipes
- The lead sulphide (PbS) formed by hydrogen sulphide (H S) and lead imparts "blue line" in the gum, along the edges of teeth and gray colour to intestinal mucosa and faeces.
- Hydrogen sulphide is derived from the putrefaction of food particles by bacteria.

Argyria

- Argyria is deposition of silver as finely granular albuminate in therapy. There is grayish blue discolouration of skin and conjunctiva and internal organs.
- The pigment is extracellular and deposited in the cementic substances like dermis, arterioles and venules. This is a permanent blemish and not harmful.

Asbestosis

Inhalation of asbestos particles leads to asbestosis and results into interstitial fibrosis

Asbestosis leads to mesothelioma in human beings.

Microscopicallly, ferruginous bodies were seen in the parenchyma. Ferruginous bodies are believed to be formed by macrophages that have phagocytozed and attempted to digest the fibers

Siderosis

- Inhalation of iron dust materials can lead to siderosis and occurs commonly in horses, mules and dogs.
- Macroscopically, brown or rusty red pigmentation can be seen.

- Microscopically, brown or black coloured irregularly shaped granules as spherical masses with in the macrophages

Endogenous pigments

- Melanin
- Lipofuchsin
- Ceroid
- Haemoglobin, haemosiderin, porphyrin.
- Haemosiderin
- Porphyrin

Melanin

- Melanin (G. Melas-Black) is a black pigment produced by oxidation of tyrosine to dihydroxy phenyl alanine by the copper containing enzyme tyrosinase in the melanocyte.
- The melanocytes are generally present in the basal layer of epidermis, retina, iris and pia-arachnoid of black animals and in the oral mucosa (Jersey cows).
- Lower vertebrates, it is widespread in different tissues.
- In lower animals, melanin have protective effect in inflammation.
- The melanin pigment protects from ultraviolet radiation.
- Pathologically, hypo/ hyper-pigmentation may occur in animals.

Melanin

Melanin is genetically controlled, high-molecular-weight bichrome compound protein.

Melanin is iron and sulphur containing brownish granular pigment, very minute, uniformly regular, spherical granules. It may be black, brown or red depending on the amount and distribution.

Types of melanin

Eumelanin: Black-brown insoluble pigment

Phaeomelanin: Light-coloured sulphur containing pigment in some avian and mammalian species and in human red haired people.

Melanin synthesis

Skin-Stratum germinativum-Basal cell layer

↓

Neural crests-Peculiar branching cells-Derived and migrate

↓

Melanoblasts

↓

Tyrosinase
(Copper protein enzyme)

↓

Tyrosine (dihydroxy phenylalanine) by oxidation and converted into

↓

Dioxyphenylalanine (DOPA) and

↓

Melanin (Dopaquinone)
(In melanocyte, tyrosinase accumulate in Golgi apparatus called premelanomse and becomes melanosomes as melanin polymer depending on protein frame work)

↓

Dispersed to other cells

↓

By macrophages
(Called melanophores i.e. carriers of melanin; Macrophages cannot produce melanin as the lack tyrosinase)

↓

Transport and deposit to other parts of the body

Tyrosine is precursor for

1. Melanin
2. Adrenaline
3. Thyroxin
4. Adrenal hormones
5. Melatonin

Increased pigmentation of skin may be

- Generalized

- Localized

May be caused by

- Diseases
- Idiopathic

Hypopigmentation: "Too less production of melanin"

Copper deficiency in cattle and sheep results in loss of coat colour.

Albinism: Depigmentation seen in copper deficiency, sulphur containing compounds like thiouracil combine with copper and makes it unavailable for tyrosinase and sulfhydryl group also causes above effect.

- Melanin deficiencies due to lack of tyrosinase.
- The melanocytes appear normal. Lack of pigmentation in skin, hair, sclera or iris on exposure to sunlight may lead to development of skin cancer.

Leukoderma is a condition in which local loss of skin pigments which is likely to be seen in the collar, saddle or harness.

Vitiligo is partial or complete loss of melanocytes in the epidermis.
Hyperpigmentation "Too much production of melanin"

- The condition is found in melanomas and occasionally in malignant melanomas.
- White/ Gray horses are susceptible to melanomas. Naevus (pigmented moles) is seen in human beings commonly.
- Focal accumulation of pigments occurs in mammary gland and surrounding fat in gilts and sows.

Melanosis is a hyperpigmented area sometimes found in the intestine, (melanosis coli), heart, lung, kidney etc.

- Melanosis of cornea may lead to blindness in some breeds of dogs e.g. Boxers, Western Terriers. The condition is bilateral and symmetrical.

Hyperpigmentation of skin (*Acanthosis nigricans*) may be associated with chronic injury and hyperadrenalism.

- The melanocytes contain melanosomes having the pigment. The macrophages laden with melanin are termed as melanophores.
- Tyrosine is source of melanin, adrenaline and thyroxine

DOPA test

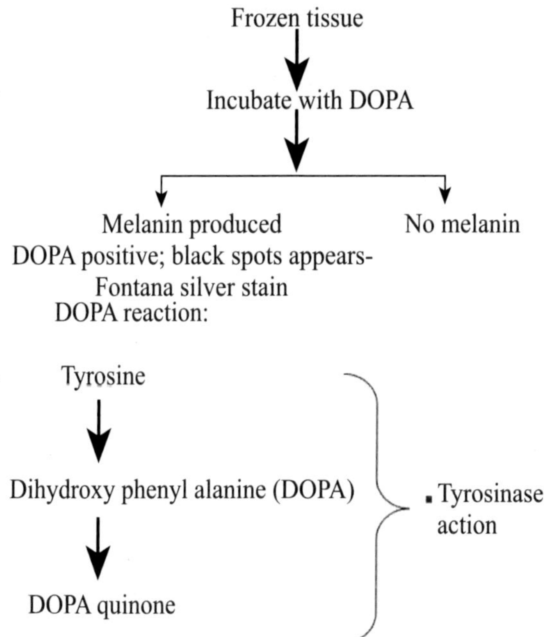

- Tissue containing melanocytes convert DOPA to DOPA quinine are tested DOPA positive while melanophores give a DOPA negative test.

Lipofuscin-Ceroid

- **Lipofuscin** (L. Fuscus-Brown) is known as '**aging pigment**' or '**wear and tear pigment**' or '**biologic garbage**'. They are brownish yellow pigments and are accumulated in post-mitotic cells like neurons, cardiomyocytes, skeletal myocytes and in slowly dividing cells like glial cells and hepatocytes. The pigment is intracellular.This pigment cannot be removed by lysosomal degradation or exocytosis. The pigment is a complex of lipid and protein derived from oxidation of polyunsaturated lipids derived from free radical injury and lipid peroxidation. They are referred to as **residual bodies** representing indigestible residues of autophagic vacuoles. The tissue discoloration is known as 'brown atrophy'.
- **Histochemistry:** Fat soluble dyes, acid fast, PAS-positive.

Ceroid is a pathological pigment

Ceroid is an early form of lipofuscin containing partially oxidised polymerised unsaturated fatty acids.

- It has got similar chemical component to lipofuscin and occurs in response to severe malnutrition including hypovitaminosis E, cancer cachexia, irradiation and inherited neuronal ceroid lipofuscinosis.
- The pigment accumulates in Kupffer cells, hepatocytes, skeletal and smooth muscle myocytes. This pigment has a deleterious effect on the cell.
- Occasionally, the pigments are seen in the small intestine of dogs called intestinal lipofuscinosis and in nutritional panniculitis in cats, minks, foals and pigs (hypovitaminosis E).
- In cats it is also due to ingestion of fish products which contains highly concentrated unsaturated fatty acids.
- Hepatic ceroidosis: Salmons and cat fish fed with rancid diets

Grossly, lipofuscin pigment gives a brown discolouration to heart and skeletal muscle and thyroid. Lipofuscin in the presence of UV light produces brown fluorescence e.g. thyroid

Microscopically, light golden brown to dark brown pigments are seen around the perinuclear areas of neurons and different myocytes. This pigment may also be extracellular (feline panniculitis) e.g. autosomal recessive- English Setter dogs

Haemosiderosis

- Haemosiderin is a golden yellow to brown granular crystalline pigments derived from hemoglobin and stored in cells.
- Normally hemosiderin is present greatest amount in spleen of horse and least in spleen of dog.
- Haemosiderosis is deposition of haemosiderin in many tissues and organs.

Haemosiderosis

- Systemic changes
- Localised changes

Causes

- Increased absorption of dietary iron
- Impaired iron utilisation
- Excess haemolysis
- Blood transfusion (Exogenous iron load)
- These are occuring as systemic derangement in chronic passive hyperaemia involving lungs where haemorrhages are seen.
- Erythrocytes are lysed and the haemosiderin is phagocytosed and deposited in the lung.
- Haemosiderin laden macrophages are called **heart failure cells**. This along with increased fibrosis gives the lung hardness and brown discolouration.
- This is referred to as **brown induration of lung**.
- Haemosiderin can also accumulate locally in haemorrhages known as localised haemosiderosis. e.g. Bruises.
- A local haemorrhage impart different colours as the wound ages. First it appears red blue.
- Haemosiderin formed from lysed RBCs are taken by macrophages, red blue colour becomes green blue (Biliverdin formation).
- Then golden yellow colour haemosiderin deposits.

Microscopically

- Haemosiderin pigments is found in cellular cytoplasm appearing as coarse, granular yellow pigment.
- Histochemically, it appears blue from prussian blue reaction.
- It is an insoluble blue black ferric ferrocyanide.

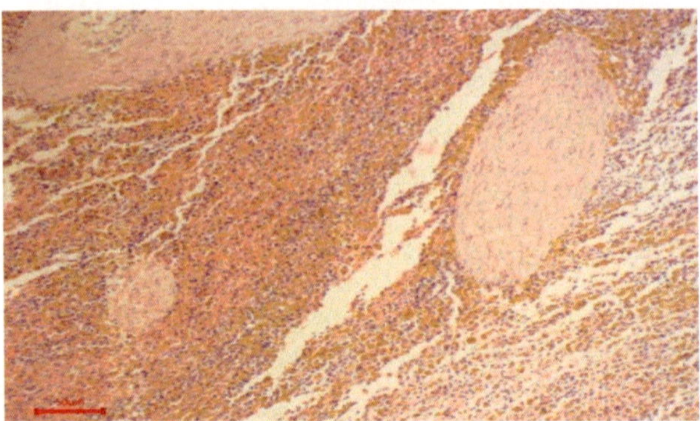

Spleen-Haemosiderosis -Golden yellow pigment in macrophage

Haemochromatosis

- This condition is due to extreme accumulation of iron in diseases. e.g. Human - Diabetes mellitus associated with hepatic fibrosis.
- In this iron overload disorder, the iron content may reach 50-60 g when compared to 2 - 3 times more than normal in adult .
- Animals - This may occur due to excessive dietary iron absorption and injection of iron

Porphyria

Porphyrin is normally present in haemoglobin, myoglobin and cytochromes. Higher pigmentation can occur due to genetic derangement or acquired based on clinical and biochemical characters. These may be congenital, erythropoietic defect, erythrohepatic protoporphyria, acute intermittent, porphyria cutanea tarda, mixed porphyria and coproporphyria.

Congenital deficiency of enzymes uroporphyrinogen II cosynthetase in human and cattle unable to use porphyrin to synthesize protoporphyrin and heme. Porphyrins use and metabolism are affected. There may be skin lesions and excessive excretion of porphyrin into faeces (Hereditary, non- symptomatic sometimes nerve lesions reported).

Jaundice in animals

Jaundice (French – yellow: icterus - Greek – jaundice). Jaundice is not a disease, it is a sign.

- Jaundice is defined as yellow discolouration of skin, sclerae, mucous membranes and internal organs caused by an increase in bilirubin concentration in tissues.

- To understand jaundice, it is essential to know the bilirubin production. Jaundice- Icteric- Subcutis

Synthesis of bile

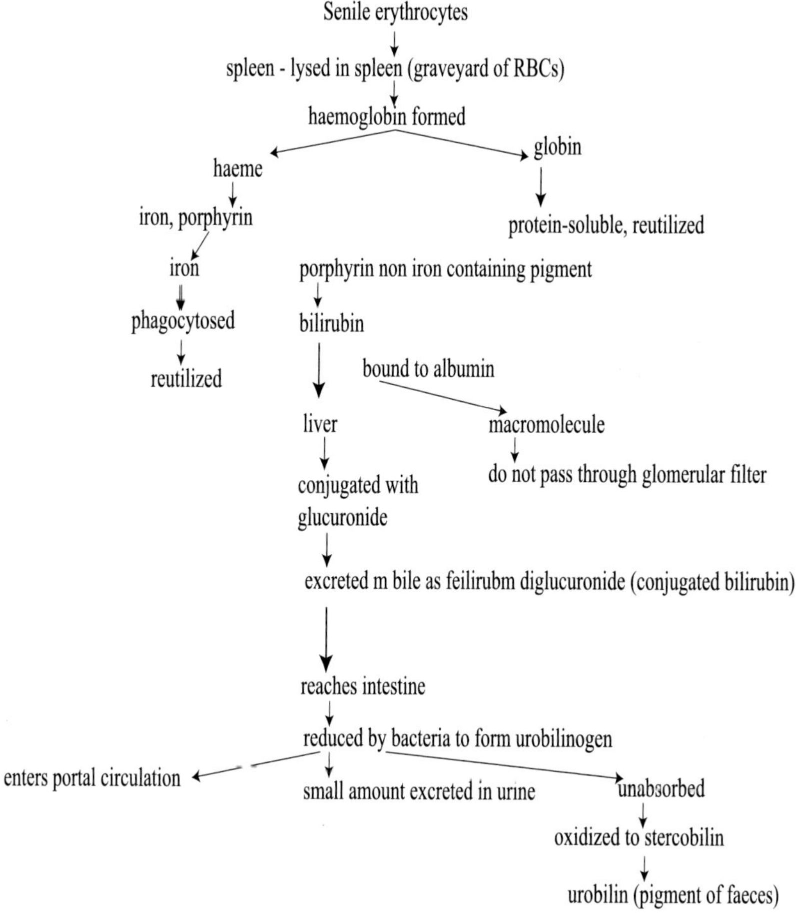

Causes of jaundice

1. Overproduction of bilirubin due to increased haemolysis.
2. Reduced uptake in liver, impaired conjugation (lack of enzymes)
3. Impaired intrahepatic secretion due to hepatic damage, intrahepatic cholestasis due to biliary obstruction
4. Impaired extrahepatic secretion due to obstruction - Due to bileduct obstruction.

Jaundice is classified into

1. Haemolytic or prehepatic jaundice
2. Toxic or intrahepatic jaundice
3. Obstructive or posthepatic jaundice

1. Haemolytic or Prehepatic Jaundice

Causes

Bacteria : *Clostridium haemolyticum*, Leptospirosis

Virus : Equine infectious anaemia

Protozoa: Babesiosis, Anaplasmosis, Haemobartonellosis, Trypanosomosis Nutritional : Phosphorus deficiency - Post parturient haemoglobinuria Phytotoxins : Resin, Saponin

Animal toxin : Snake venom

Chemicals : Copper, selenium toxicity in sheep

Icterus neonatarum, incompatible blood supply

Pathogenesis

- Excessive haemolysis results in production of greater amount of unconjugated bilirubin.
- Since there is a rate limiting, all unconjugated bilirubin cannot be converted to conjugated bilirubin.
- Hence, some amount is left in the blood. Since large amount of conjugated bilirubin is formed, it stains faeces yellow.
- When excess quantity of urobilin is formed (faeces intense yellow colour) and is also responsible for abnormal intense yellow urine.

2. Toxic or Intrahepatic Jaundice

Causes

Bacteria: Leptospirosis, Salmonellosis Virus : Infectious canine hepatitis Phytotoxins: Senecio, crotalaria

Chemicals: Phosphorus, chronic copper poisoning, chloroform, carbon tetrachloride.

Pathogenesis

- When heptocytes are necrosed, the liver is not able to convert normally formed unconjugated bilirubin.
- Since the degenerated cells are swollen and disorganised and biliary capillaries are blocked, conjugated bilirubin escapes/spills into sinusoids and enters general circulation and excreted through urine.
- Hence, blood contains both conjugated and unconjugated bilirubin

3. Obstructive or Posthepatic Jaundice

Causes

1. Blocking of bileduct from within
    - *Ascaris lumbricoides* in swine
    - *Thysanosoma astiniodes* (fringed tape worm)
    - *Fasciola gigantica* in cattle
    - Gall stones
2. Pressure on bile duts from outside

- Tumours, abscesses, granulomas, fibrosis, enlarged pancreas or lymph nodes

3. Inflammatory processes in biliary system
    - Cholangitis, cholecystitis – fascioliasis, *Dicrocoelium dendriticum*
4. Closure of bile duct orifice in duodenum
    - Duodenitis – thickening of mucosa

Pathogenesis

- The obstruction to normal flow of bile results in regurgitation of bile.
- In this case, the production of conjugated and unconjugated bilirubin is normal.
- Biliary stasis occurs due to (extra hepatic cholestasis) pressure, worms, inflammation and duodenitis.
- No urobilinogen is formed since bile is not entering to intestine.
- Faeces greasy and grey colour due to failure of fat emulsification and lack of faecal pigment. Urine is not containing urobilin.

- Steatorrhoea (Fat is faeces-undigested)and foul smelling faeces
- Clotting defects will occur due to failure of obstruction of vitamin K which is required for prothrombin formation.

Chemical Test for Bilirubin

• van den Bergh test

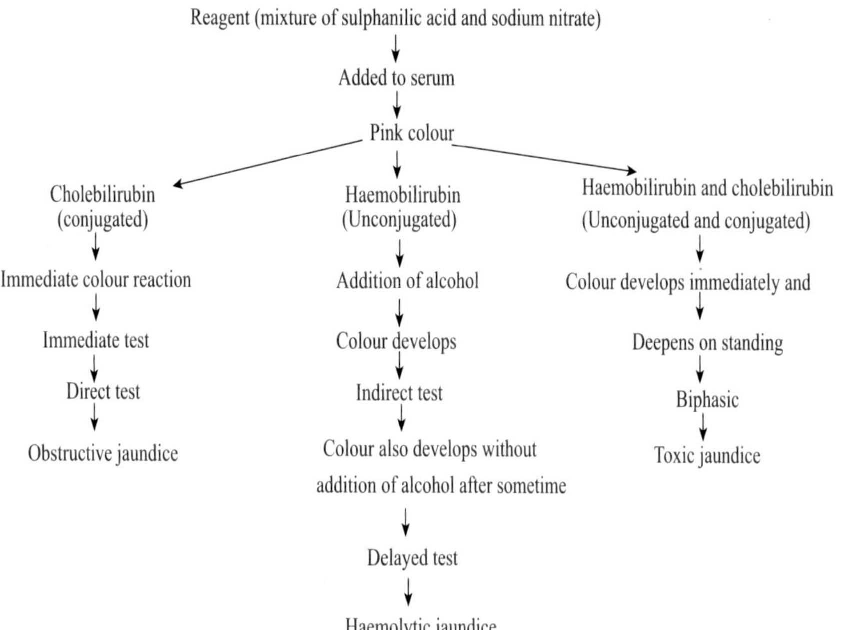

Differential Diagnosis of Jaundice

S.No.	Parameters	Haemolytic	Toxic	Hepatic
1.	Bilirubin	Increased unconjugated bilirubin	Increased conjugated and unconjugated bilirubin	Increased conjugated bilirubin
2.	Serum van den Bergh test	Indirect	Biphasic	Direct
3.	Urine bilirubin	Not present	Present	Present
4.	Urine urobilinogen	Slightly present	Present	Not present
5.	Feaces	Intense yellow, no smell	Normal	Clay coloured, greasy, foul smelling
6.	Liver function tests	Negative	Positive	Negative

S.No.	Parameters	Haemolytic	Toxic	Hepatic
7.	Blood prothrombin time	Normal	Prolonged	Prolonged
8.	Total serum cholesterol	Normal	Decreased	Increased
9.	Haemoglobinuria, anaemia and blood parasite	Present	Absent	Absent

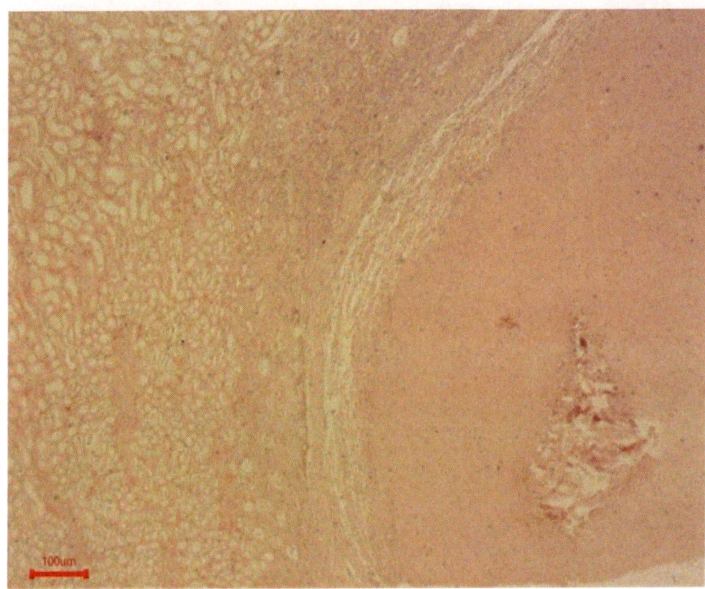

Dystrophic Calcification-Lung-Tuberculosis

9

Photosensitization

Photosensitization is activation of photodynamic chemicals on the skin by long wave length UV or occasionally by visible light

- Necrosis and edema are produced in the exposed areas of skin of animals.
- The cellular damage by photosensitization is due to release of reactive oxygen species leading to mast cell degranulation and production of chemical mediators of inflammation.

Factors Necessary for Photosensitization in Animals

- Oxygen
- Sunlight
- Photodynamic chemicals
- Skin devoid of hair or wool and lacking pigments

Types of Photosensitization

1. Type I: Primary photosensitization
2. Type II: Abnormal porphyrin metabolism associated photosensitization
3. Type III: Hepatogenous photosensitization

1. Type I: Primary Photosensitization Causes

Plants containing helianthrones (e.g. hypericine in *Hypericum perforatum*; fagopyrin in *Fagopyrum esculentum*) and furocoumarin pigments (e.g. *Cymopterus watsonii* and *Ammi majus*), tetracyclines and sulphonamides

Examples

- Phytotoxins from furocoumarin plants exposed to fungi or other injury may be absorbed into skin which reacts with UV light

- Phenothiazine is converted into photoreactive compound when bypasses the liver, reaches the skin causing photodermatitis on exposure to sunlight

2. Type II: Abnormal Porphyrin Metabolism Associated Photosensitization

- Due to inherited enzyme deficiency, abnormal porphyrin photodynamic metabolic products like uroporphyrin and protoporphyrin accumulate in blood and tissues.
- The uroporphyrin also causes discoloration of bone known as "**osteohaemochromatosis**" and teeth called "**pink teeth**".

Examples

- Bovine congenital porphyria
- Bovine haematopoietic protoporphyria

3. Type III: Hepatogenous Photosensitization

Hepatogenous photosensitization is caused by impaired hepatic capacity to excrete phylloerythrin derived from chlorophyll degradation in the alimentary tract, mainly affecting herbivores.

Causes

- Hepatocellular damage or injury (Toxic hepatitis due to *Lantana camara*, *Tribulus terrestris*, plants producing pyrrolizidine alkaloids, sporidesmins)
- Inherited hepatic defects
- Biliary obstruction
- Infection: Leptospirosis
- Chemicals: CCl_4 poisoning

Gross pathology

Hairless, non-pigmented skin exposed to sun light (Horses: face, nose, distal extremities; Cattle: teats, udder, perineum, nose; Sheep: pinnae, eyelids, face, nose, coronary band with heavy fleece, facial eczema or "swollen head"), erythema, edema, blisters, exudation, necrosis and sloughing of necrotic tissue.

Histopathology

- Coagulative necrosis of epidermis, subepidermal vesiculation, swelling of endothelial cells, fibrinoid degeneration and thrombosis of blood vessels leading to edema.
- Secondary bacterial infection culminate in sloughing of epidermis and adnexae.

10

The Disturbances of Growth

The Disturbances of Growth

- The disturbances in growth cover a broader spectrum of changes from no growth (Aplasia) to uncontrolled growth (Neoplasia).
- While uncontrolled growth (neoplasm) is not dealt here, the other forms of growth disturbances are considered in this chapter.

Cellular Adaptation to Injury

- The cells respond to altered physiological or pathological stimuli by adapting themselves.
- These changes are reflected as atrophy, hyperplasia, hypertrophy, metaplasia and dysplasia besides aplasia and hypoplasia.
- Following an injurious stimulus or to stress, the normal cell's homeostatic state may respond with cellular injury and death or adapt itself.
- Hence, the cellular adaptation to the increased demand is a state in between normal and stressed and injured cell.
- Cells may fail to develop or adapt to changing environment or physiological or pathological stimuli.

These are

1. Aplasia and Agenesis
2. Hypoplasia
3. Atrophy
4. Hyperplasia
5. Hypertrophy
6. Pseudohypertropgy

7. Metaplasia
8. Dysplasia
9. Neoplasia

1. Aplasia and Agenesis

Agenesis is without beginning

Aplasia (Gr. A: Without; not; Plasia: Development; formation) is the complete failure of an organ to develop. Organ may be totally absent.

- This development disturbance occurs in the embryo or foetus in utero.
- In the place of the organ, rudimentary tissue of fat and connective tissue are present.
- The condition is incompatible with life, death occurs, when it involves vital organs like heart, brain and lung tissue etc.

2. Hypoplasia "Do not develop to full size"

- It is the failure of an organ or tissue to attain its full normal adult size.

Causes may be genetic or non-genetic

- Any injury occurring in late stages of development of fetus or neonates. e.g. Genetic mutation affects proper differentiation and migration of cells in embryo, virus causes hypoplastic changes e.g. Bovine Viral Diarrhoea in calf, Feline Pan Leukopenia virus, Feline Infectious Peritonitis, and Feline spongiform encephalopathy in cat causes cerebellar hypoplasia; drug induced hypoplasia e.g. Teratogens (Valproic acid (VPA) causes cerebellar hypoplasia in rats and ferrets) occurs through degeneration and necrotic changes.
- Pathological changes: - Organ will be smaller than adult size. The cells show alterations in lysosomes and inspissated protein in cytoplasm. The phagolysosomes increase in size with lipofuscin pigment.

3. Atrophy "Cells are not dead but have diminished fucntions"

- Atrophy is the decrease in the size (quantitative) or amount (numerical) of cells/tissues/organ after attaining full normal growth.
- Atrophy is representing adaptation to deficient nutrient supply, lack of stimulation and decreased work load. This may affect any organ or part of an organ.

- Atrophy can be broadly classified as physiological atrophy and pathological atrophy.

i. Physiological atrophy

a) **Involution of the organs** can be observed as the age is advanced. Involution is the decrease in the size of the organ due to decrease in the number of cells, caused by apoptosis.

   e.g. Involution of thymus on attaining puberty, uterine involution after parturition (decrease in smooth muscle size and number)

(b) **Senile atrophy**: Atrophy of the organs occurs with ageing and reproductive organs like testis and ovaries are the first to show such changes. It is associated with loss of cells.

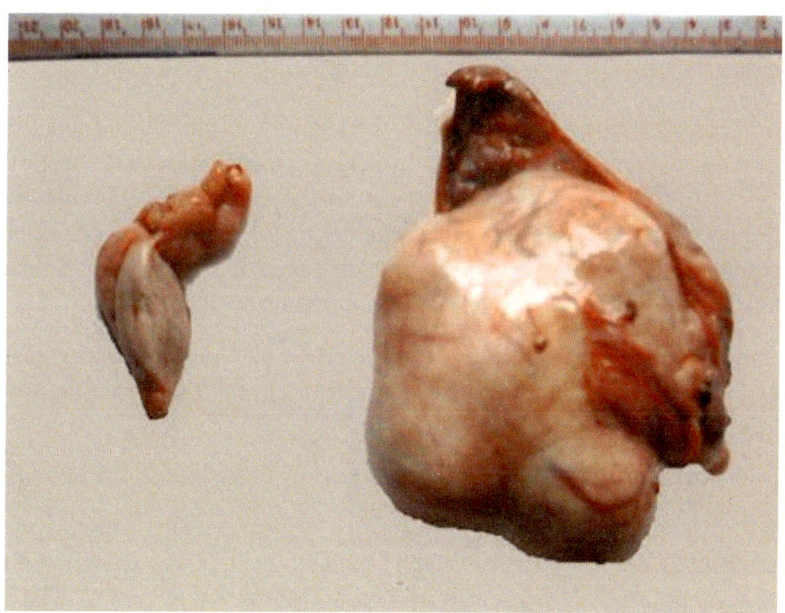

Testicles –Atrophy; Right-Tumour; Left-Atrophy

ii. Pathological Atrophy

(a) **Nutritional atrophy:** This is due to starvation. Starvation of the tissue is caused by malnutrition, malabsorption, chronic infection, parasitism, neoplasia etc.

   Mismothering is also quoted in starvation atrophy in neonates. In starvation following depletion of glycogen and fat reserves, protein of the musculature and vital organs is lost, resulting in muscular wasting.

(b) **Angiotrophic atrophy:** Diminished blood supply (ischaemia, chronic passive congestion, anaemia) may lead to atrophic changes.

e.g. Parasitic ischaemia caused by *Strongylus* larvae by the occlusion of femoral artery leads to atrophy of hind limb in horses.

Hepatic atrophy can occur due to decreased portal venous blood flow.

Chronic venous congestion results in centrilobular necrosis of liver due to inadequate oxygen and nutrition supplied to the hepatocytes.

(c) **Disuse atrophy**

i. **Decreased work load**: Decrease in the size of the body musculature due to inactivity as in the case of race horses.

ii. **Immobilization**: Skeletal muscle atrophic changes can occur in plaster casted animals.

In fracture, there will be decrease in the size of the cells or myocytes.

(d) **Neurotrophic atrophy:** Decrease in the size of muscle fibres occurs if a nerve is severed or injured. e.g. In horses, laryngeal muscle atrophy occurs due to the injury to left recurrent laryngeal nerve (**snoring**-Hemiplegia-Paralysis of left recurrent laryngeal nerve) and shoulder muscle atrophy (**sweeny**) occurs due to suprascapular nerve injury affecting supraspinatus, infraspinatus and triceps muscles.

(e) **Pressure atrophy:** In space occupying lesions like tumours, abscesses, cysts etc., the neighbouring tissues undergo atrophic changes mainly due to lack of nutrition from pressure ischemia.

(f) **Endocrine atrophy**: Prolonged steroid therapy leads to atrophy of zona fasciculata of the adrenal gland.

Castration leads to atrophy of prostate. Hyperestrogenism associated with sertoli cell tumour results in seminiferous cell atrophy. Ovariectomy leads to uterine atrophy. Thyroid atrophy can occur in reduced TSH, idiopathic autoimmune disease.

Pathogenesis

In atrophy, the cells survive and are smaller in size with decreased function. There is imbalance between protein synthesis and degradation or loss protein. That is excessive protein loss degradation overproduction of proteins. Atrophy and atrophic changes can be attributed to autophagocytosis and heterophagocytosis with destruction of cytoplasmic organelles like ribosomes, mitochondria and lysosomes and by ubiquitin-proteasome pathway wherein the proteins combine with ubiquitin, a cytosolic peptide and then it is destroyed (that is called proteasome). Glucocorticoid and thyroid hormone stimulate proteasome mediated protein destruction. Insulin has opposite effect. Cytokines, TNF and IL-1/IL-3 signally accelerate the muscle proteolysis by their pathway.

Morbid/ Gross Changes

Affected organs show decreased weight and volume, wrinkling of surface membrane and tortuous blood vessels too large for the volume of the tissue. Organs may be fibrosed and become firm. Fat shows serous atrophy (indicating starvation) i.e. clear/yellowish gelatinous material is seen in place of fat especially cardiac fat, renal fat etc.The organ may become soft and flabby and loss of tone and tissue colour.

Microscopic Changes

Cells are smaller than normal and decrease in number. Looks as too many nucleated cells in a field. No mitosis. Sometimes, complete disappearance of the cells is found. Adipocytes become smaller. Interstitial hyaluronic acid and mucopolisacharides are increased. Sometimes brown atrophy is encountered. Brownish discolouration is due to the membrane bound, indigested residual bodies in the cytoplasm. Autophagic vacuoles as residual bodies in lipofuscin granules. Ultra structurally, there will be reduction in organelles.

4. Hyperplasia 'Quantitative increase in number of cells'

Hyperplasia is the increase in the size of the tissue or an organ or a part of an organ due to quantitative increase in the number of cells.

Hyperplasia classification

i. Physiological hyperplasia

ii. Pathological hyperplasia

i. Physiological hyperplasia

(a) Physiological hyperplasia may be the result of hormonal influence as in the case of increase in the size of mammary gland due to glandular epithelial cell proliferation in puberty and pregnancy.

(b) Compensatory hyperplasia

- It occurs due to partial loss of hepatocytes in liver.
- Hepatic regeneration occurs following partial hepatectomy by the proliferation of surviving cells.
- These cells are primed from the matrix degradation products followed by proliferation under the influence of growth factors (HGF) and cytokines (TNF-α, IL-6 . EGF, TGF-α etc.) and aided by adjuvants like norepinephrine and growth inhibition influenced by TGF-β, (Growth factors), with reduction in the growth factors and adjuvants.
- Compensatory hyperplasia can also be observed in abraded epidermis in which basal layer proliferates to form the superficial layers.

ii. Pathological hyperplasia: This is most commonly caused by excessive hormonal stimulation. e.g. endometrial hyperplasia or effects of growth factors on target cells. In canine uterus, cystic endometrial hyperplasia occurs in prolonged progesterone secretion; in wound healing, hyperplasia of connective tissue (e.g. fibroblast and blood vessels) occurs under the influence of growth factors; hyperplasia also occurs in viral infections involving the epithelium i.e. epidermis or mucosal epithelium. e.g. papilloma virus infections. Pathological hyperplasia may also lead to cancerous growth.

- Pathological hyperplasia may be localized or generalized/diffused.
- Localized hyperplasia - e.g. Nodular hyperplasia in liver, spleen of aged dogs.
- Generalized/diffused hyperplasia- e.g. diffuse enlargement of an organ, prostatic hyperplasia in dogs and thymus hyperplasia in case of goiter.

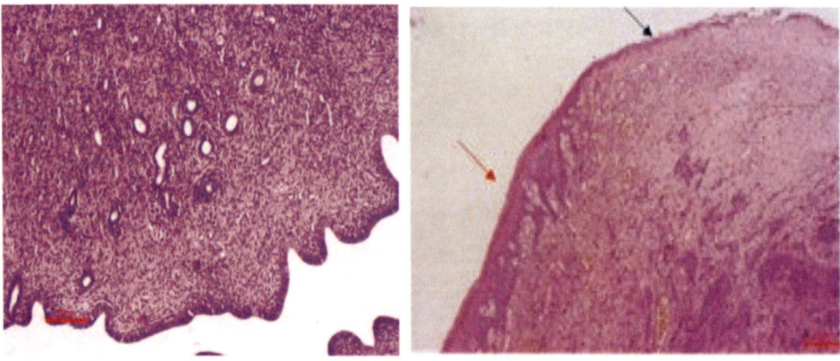

Mucosal hyperplasia- Uterus; Normal (Blue arrow); Hyperplasia (Red arrow)

Hyperplastic ability depends on different adult cell types

Accordingly three cell populations are identified: based on mitotic capacity

1. **Labile cells:** These cells can proliferate normally and continuously. e.g. Epidermis, bone marrow cells
2. **Stable cells:** These cells proliferate when need arises. e.g. Liver, bone, cartilage, smooth muscle
3. **Permanent cells:** These cells have lost their ability to regenerate/ become hyperplastic. e.g. Neurons, cardiac and skeletal myocytes.

5. Hypertrophy

- It is the increase in the size of the cells or the organ. The number of the cells does not increase. The hypertrophic changes are seen in the permanent/stable cells. Striated muscles are most commonly affected.
- In microscopic view, the organ will be normal but the cells are bigger.

The number and the size of the organelles will be increased due to the increase in the functional demand. e.g. smooth endoplasmic reticulum in hepatocytes are enlarged in chronic alcoholism and increase in the size of the rough endoplasmic reticulum and Golgi apparatus as a need for increased synthesis of proteins (e.g. collagen and immunoglobulin); the mitochondrial number varies with ATP requirements.

Types of Hypertrophy

i. **Physiologic Hypertrophy:** It occurs following work or exercise/ specific hormonal stimulus. e.g. Muscles in race and draft horses; in pregnancy with increased estrogen stimulation hypertrophy of uterus occurs and in lactation mammary gland development occurs under the influence of prolactin and estrogen.

ii. **Compensatory Hypertrophy:** It occurs due to the loss of a part of the organ or loss of one of the paired organs (One kidney undergoes hypertrophy with the loss of the other) or due to the obstruction of the lumen in hollow muscular organ (Right ventricular hypertrophy in pulmonary stenosis).With the continued haemodynamic overload, the compensatory mechanisms fail, resulting in the decompensation and cardiac failure.

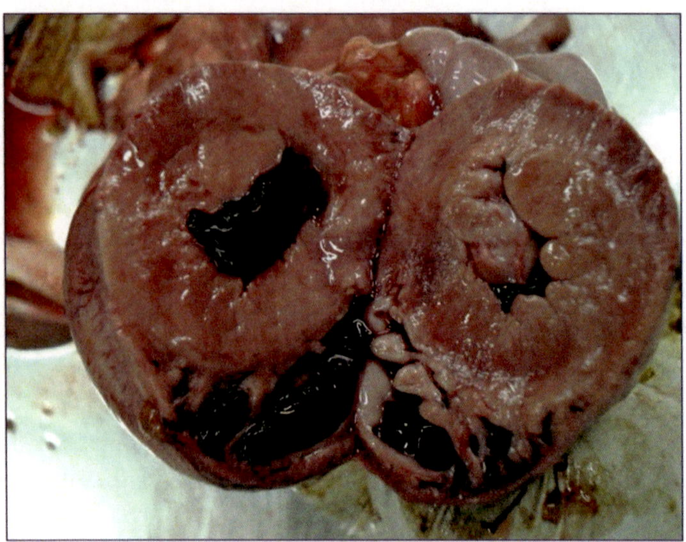

Concentric hypertrophy-Heart-Narrowing of chamber

Mechanism of hypertrophy involves many signal transduction pathways with induction of a number of genes and synthesis of cellular protein. So there will be increase in growth factors, its receptors (TGF-β, fibroblast growth factor), transcriptional factor (C- fos) and vasoactive agents especially endothelin-1.

6. Pseudohypertrophy

It is an enlargement of (increase in size) of an organ not due to primary tissue but due to increase in some other tissue like fat.

7. Metaplasia

Metaplasia is a reversible change in which one adult cell type is replaced by another adult cell type of the same germinal layer.

It is also defined as the transformation of one cell type to another cell type within the embryological limits. Metaplasia may involve epithelial or mesenchymal tissue.

In metaplasia, one type of epithelium may be converted into another, usually less special type or one type of mesenchymal tissue into another type.

While metaplasia is reversible, it is considered as a double edged sword, as it may lead to cancer.

Mechanism

Metaplasia may arise from reprogramming of stem cells (Reserve cells in epithelium) or from undifferentiated mesenchymal cells present in the connective tissue. The stem cells may differentiate following changes in signals through cytokines, growth factors and extracellular matrix. The tissue specific and differentiation genes involved are bone morphogenetic protein, TGF- β etc. that induce chondro-osteogenic expressions. Some transcription factors involved in the cellular differentiation are Myo-D for muscle, PPAR-γ for adipose tissue,and CBFA-1for osteoblast differentiation.

Metaplastic changes may be caused by chronic irritation, nutritional deficiency, neoplasm etc.

Types of Metaplasia

i. Epithelial metaplasia
ii. Mesenchymal metaplasia
iii. Mesothelial metaplasia

I. Epithelial metaplasia (Columnar to squamous type)

Squamous metaplasia: It may occur due to many reasons like chronic irritation, nutritional deficiency etc.

i. Chronic irritation from chemicals, carcinogens or other chemicals.
   a) Smoking: In lung of smokers, ciliated cuboidal and columnar epithelia of airways are converted into stratified squamous epithelium.
   b) Estrogenism: Stratified squamous metaplasia of prostate or urinary tract.
   c) Calculi: Calculi of salivary gland, biliary calculi, pancreas etc.

ii. Nutritional deficiency: Vitamin A deficiency produces squamous metaplasia of esophageal mucous glands of chicken, transitional epithelium of urinary bladder, cuboid and columnar epithelial cells lining the eye and salivary gland ducts.

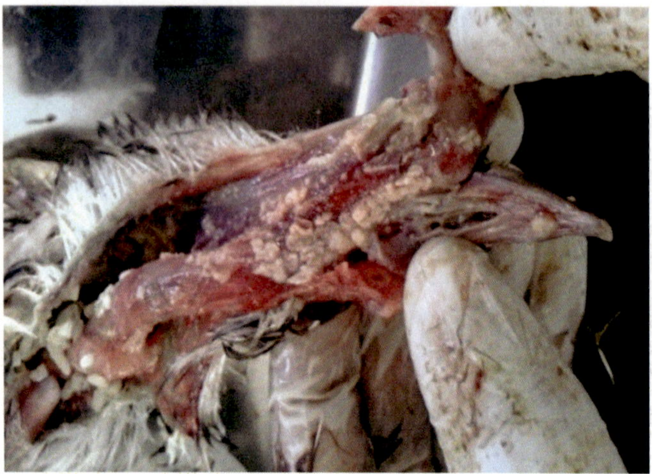

Chicken- Nutritional Roup- Hypovitaminosis A- Epithelial metaplasia

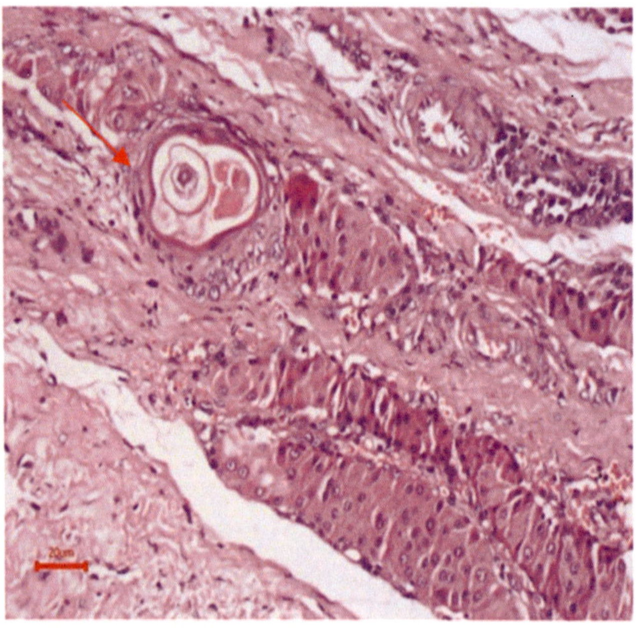

Epithelial metaplasia- Cuboidal to squamous type
(Red arrow) - Perianal gland adenocarcinoma

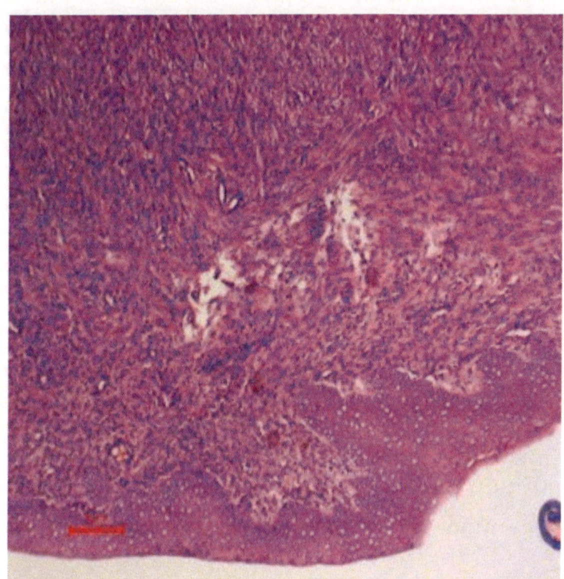

Epithelial metaplasia- Stratified squamous type-Uterine mucosa

Though the squamous metaplasia having multiple layers of epithelial cells and can be protective against an irritant. It also poses threat or disadvantages. e.g. Ciliary epithelial cell more resistance to infection and its clearance if replaced by squamous epithelial cells.

ii. Mesenchymal metaplasia

- Osseous metaplasia in injured soft tissue and metaplastic changes in mesenchymal tissue results in the formation of cartilage and bone in mixed mammary tumour of dogs and myeloid metaplasia leading to extramedullary haematopoesis in adult liver and spleen following injury to bone marrow.

iii. Mesothelial metaplasia

- Mesothelial cell lining pleura, pericardium and peritoneal layers if irritated with fluid accumulation; the flat cells are transformed into cuboidal to columnar epithelium

8. Dysplasia

- The term dysplasia is applied to the tissue malformed during maturation.
- **Definition:** There will be alteration in size, shape and orientation of tissue. The condition is mainly affecting the epithelium.

- Dysplastic changes are commonly found in the eye, skin, brain and skeletal system.
- The developmental defect involved complex interactions among three germinal layers.
- In dysplasia, there will be loss of uniformity of cells and their architecture
- It is characterized by pleomorphism (Change in the size and shape of cells), abnormally enlarged (karyomegaly) hyperchromic nuclei, increased mitosis and disorderly arranged cells.
- Dysplasia when marked and in which all layers of stratified squamous epithelium are involved, it is called 'preinvasive carcinoma' or **'Carcinoma in situ'.** The epithelial layers are haphazardly arranged and jumped to one another
- The condition is mild to moderate and reversed if the stimulus is removed.

Fibrous dysplasia: Normal bone tissue is replaced by fibrous connective tissue but the growth will not progress in tumours.

9. Neoplasia (Neo-New; Plasia-Growth)

New growth of cells, uncontrolled and serves no useful function

11

Inflammation

Definitions

Reaction of vascularised living tissue to local injury caused by various agents like microbes or necrotic tissue

Inflammation – Reaction of blood vessels

– Accumulation of fluid and leucocytes in extra vascular tissues

Inflammation and repair always go hand in hand

Beneficial effects of Inflammation

To destroy / dilute the injurious agent (microbes; toxins) and to protect cell from injury (necrosis)

Harmful Effects of Inflammation

- Chronic inflammatory reactions e.g. rheumatoid arthritis
- Atherosclerosis
- Pulmonary fibrosis
- Hypersensitivity reactions
- Insect bites
- Drugs, toxins

Repair produces scars that causes mechanical obstruction and loss of functions

Types of inflammation based on duration

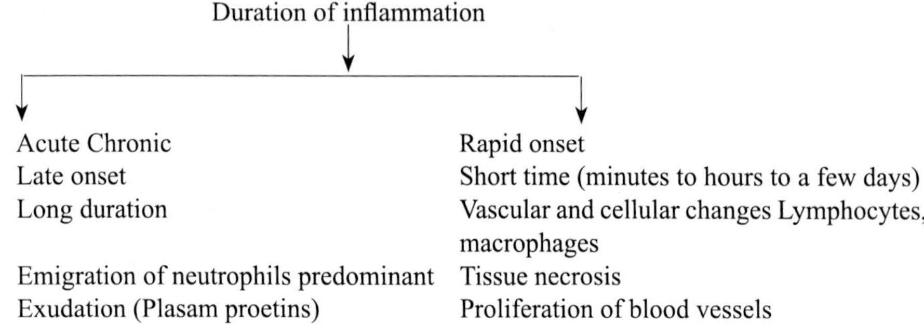

Cardinal Signs of Inflammation

There are five important local signs of inflammation.

First four of them were described in first century (AD35) by the Italian scientist

Cornelius Celsus.

Rudolf Virchow (AD 858), the German pathologist added the fifth sign.

Cardinal signs are mainly attributed to vascular changes at the site of inflammation.

The cardinal signs are

1. **Red (L. Rubor): -** It is due to the increased supply of blood (hyperemia) to the area of inflammation.
2. **Swelling (L. Tumour):** - It is due to the increased blood flow, adding volume to the tissue and exudates into the inflammatory area.
3. **Heat (L. Calor):** - It is due to the increased blood supply to area of inflammation carrying warm blood from the interior of the body and increased rate of metabolism at the site of inflammation leading to increased production of heat.
4. **Pain (L. Dolor):** - Pain in the area of inflammation is due to the increased pressure on sensory nerve endings and stretching of tissue due to accumulation of exudates.
5. **Loss of function (L. Functio laeso) :-** The affected part looses its function due to swelling, pain and tissue destruction.

Acute inflammation

Acute Inflammation is a vascular response to cell and tissue injury by various agents (Physical, chemical, biological).

Objectives

i. to kill, degrade, remove or dilute the causes of injury

ii. to phagocytose and remove debris

iii. to repair the damaged caused, so as the affected tissue returns to normal structure and functions.

Aetiology (Causes) of Inflammation

- Infectious agents – bacteria, fungi, virus etc.
- Chemical agents – acids, alkalies etc.
- Physical agents – burns, electricity, radiation, cold
- Environmental chemicals
- Venom (snake, insect)
- Immunological reactions – Ag – Ab reactions hypersensitivity) (Type-I to IV
- Nutritional imbalances – vitamins, minerals
- Necrotic tissue

Basics and Usefulness of Acute Inflammation

Progress and purpose of acute inflammation

Three phases of progression

i. Fluidic phase (Exudative)

ii. Cellular phase

iii. Reparative phase

Purpose of progressive phase

i. Fluidic phase

To dilute surround and contain injurious agents and damage. Limiting spread to adjacent normal tissue.

Exudation of fluid and protein (albumin, fibrinogen) increased vascular permeability (due to injury) and chemical molecules (cause damage indirectly).

Chemical molecules (mediators)

a. Initiate and facilitate the recruitment and movement of neutrophils through capillary wall into injured tissue

b. Form "directional concentration gradient" (highest at the source and lowest at the periphery,) function as chemoattractant/molecules. Migrating neutrophils to entrap inciting stimulus

ii. **Cellular phase**

To kill and /or digest the agent, limit extent and severity of injury and end the provoked microvascular response. These also injured adjacent normal tissue to varying extent and degree

iii. **Reparative phase**

Injury also stimulates tissues to release molecules.

Characteristic is migration of macrophages and removing the injurious agent. These cells also release molecules involved in tissue repair. If tissue loss is minimal, re-epithelialization and supporting stroma occurs. If extensive damage occurs the reparative process involves neovascularization, granulation tissue formation, re-epithelization and scar tissue formation (scarring, reparative fibrosis).

Sequential Events in Acute Inflammation

Vascular Changes in Acute Inflammation

Julius Cohnheim (1839 – 1884)

1. Changes in Blood Vessels following Injury (tissue damage, microbial virulence factors, etc)

- Transient/Momentary vasoconstriction of arterioles lasting for a few seconds; In mild infection, reaction disappears in 3-5 seconds. In severe injury, it lasts for several minutes.
- Vasodilation (arteriolar dilatation – nerve stimuli from axonal reflex also)
- Increased blood flow
- Opening of new capillary beds

- Brought about by substances – Histamine, chemical mediators of inflammation

2. Changes in the Rate of Flow

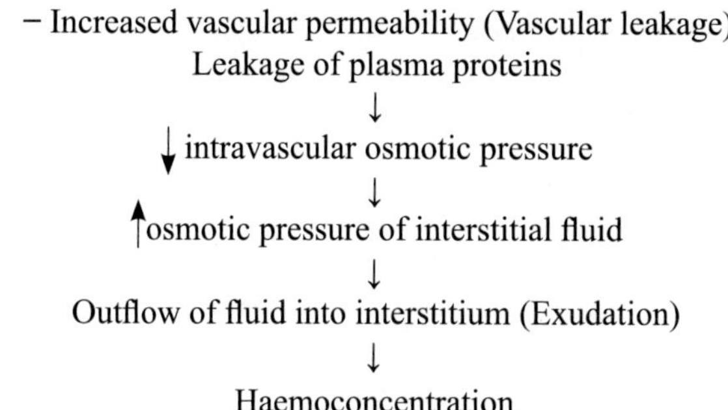

3. Essential for Movement of Leucocytes into ECF (Extracellular fluid)

a. Haemoconcentration

b. Endothelium becomes leaky

c. Activated endothelial cells release prostaglandin which causes vascular dilatation and cytokines (IL-1, TNF, TGF-β) which are chemotactic to leucocytes and procoagulants for coagulation.

Besides perivascular mast cells degranulate and release histamine which increase post capillary permeability, heparin antagonizes coagulation and angiogenic and leukotrienes which induce pain. Substance P is released by the nerve.

i. By increasing the capillary bed in the area

ii. Swelling of endothelial cells

iii. Hemoconcentration

iv. Margination of leucocytes

4. Slowing of Blood Flow – from Capillary Filing and Endothelial Swelling

- Increased vascular permeability
- Protein-rich fluid exudation
- Haemoconcentration results (Increased concentration of erythrocytes and increased viscosity).

5. Emigration of Leucocytes

- Margination of leucocytes-Fallout of circulation to reach endothelium for adhesion

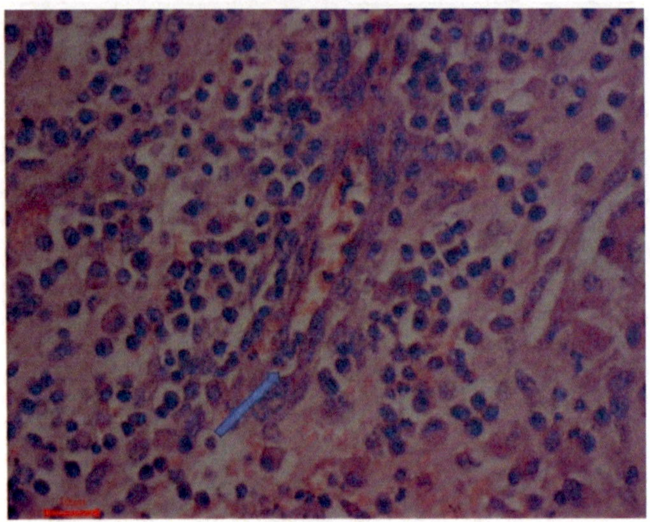

Marginatin of leucocytes (arrow)

- Rolling – selectin – selectin receptors and PEI
- Pavementing- as surface ligands increase → Leucocytes
- Adhesion- operated by integrin, ICAM
- Emigration-PECAM1 etc.
- All the above changes may take 15-30 minutes in mild injury and extend more in severe injury

Adhesion molecules		
Endothelial molecules	**Leukocyte receptors**	**Activities**
P-Selectin CD62P	Sialyl-Lewis X PSGL-1	Rolling of neutrophils, monocytes, lymphocytes
E-Selectin CD62E	Sialyl-Lewis X ESL-1, PSGL-1	Rolling, adhesion to endothelium of neutrophils, monocytes, T-Lymphocytes
ICAM-1	CD11/CD18 (Integrins) (LFA-1, MAC-21)	Adhesion, arrest, transmigration of all leukocytes
VCAM-1	α4β1 (VLA4)-Integrins α4β7 (LPAM-1)	Adhesion of eosinophils, monocytes, lymphocytes
GlyCam-1 CD34	L-Selectin	Lymphocyte homing to endothelial venules; Neutrophils, monocytes rolling

ICAM-Intercellular Adhesion Molecule; VCAM-Vascular cell Adhesion Molecule

Events in Leukocyte Activation

Chemotactic agents (Bacterial products, C5a, LTB4, IL-8) bind to specific are i to v (Nine events)

But how do these diverse chemotactic agents actually induce directed cell movement (i.e., chemotaxis)? Not all the answers are known, but several important steps and second messengers are recognized.

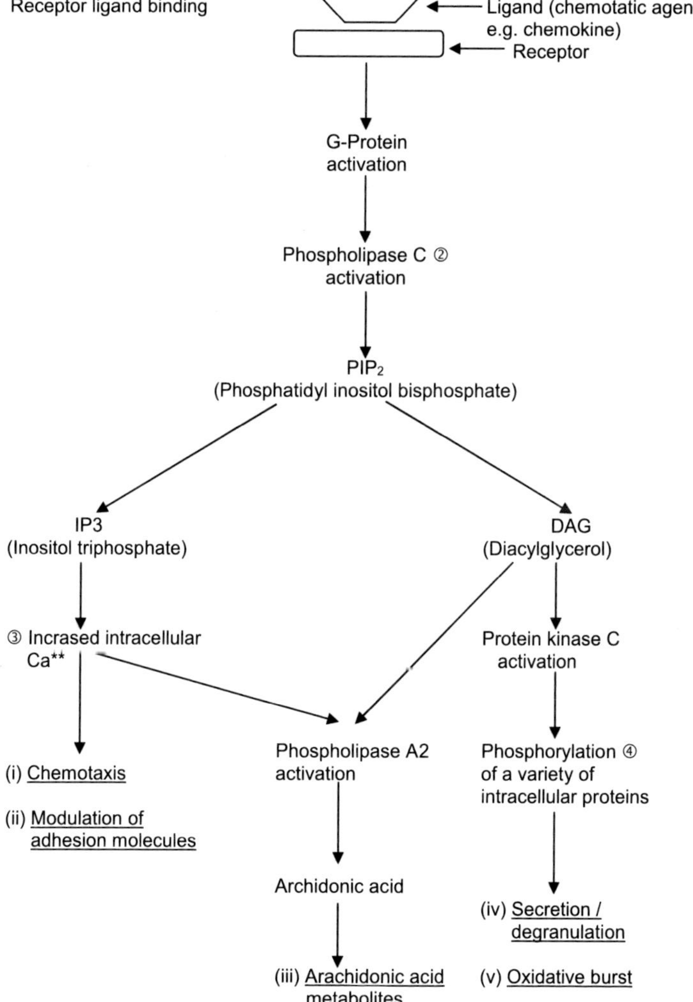

Biochemical events in leukocyte activation. The key events are : (1) receptor-ligand binding, (2) phospholipase C activation, (3) increased intracellular calcium and (4) activation of protein kinase C, resulting in protein phosphorylation. The biological activities that result from leukocyte activation include : (i) chemotaxis, (ii) modulation of adhesion molecules, (iii) elaboration of arachidonic acid metabolites, (iv) secretion / degranulation and (v) the oxidative burst.

Chemotaxis and Leukocyte Activation

Adherent leukocyte emigrates through interendothelial junction, transverse basement membrane and move forward to site of injury along a gradient chemotactic agent.

Neutrophils emigrate first -24-48h followed by monocytes and lymphocytes.

Leukocyte Activation Process

Chemotactic agents (Bacterial products, C5a, LTB4, IL-8) bind to specific receptors in leukocytes producing secondary messengers that mediate activating G-protein which in turn activates phospholipase C that split PIP2 (phosphoinositol phosphate) to IP3 (Inositol triphosphate and DAG (Diacylglycerol). IP3 causes an increase in intracellular calcium ions which are chemotactic and modulate adhesion molecules. DAG by activating protein kinase C induces phosphorylation of intracellular proteins resulting in secretion and granulation. Increased intracellular Ca+ and DAG activate phospholipase A2 which breakdown arachidonic acid to form arachidonic acid metabolites.

End results are

1. Degranulation and secretion of enzymes
2. Activation of oxidative burst
3. Production of arachidonic acid metabolites
4. Modulation of leukocyte adhesion molecules

6. Stasis

Exudation " Hall mark of acute inflammation"

Consequent to increase vascular permeability, exudation (vascular leakage) of fluid and plasma protein occur into interstitium.

Increased hydrostatic pressure or decreased osmotic pressure of blood results in escape of fluid or protein in to interstitium called exudate.

7. Diapedesis of Erythrocytes

- Movement of erythrocytes outside the blood vessel during inflammation.

Chemotaxis

- Unidirectional migration of cells towards a chemical attractant
- It is the force that attracts leucocytes into the inflamed tissue.

Chemotactic Agents

Exogenous	Endogenous
Bacterial products	Chemical mediators like C5a (complement)
	Leukotriene B4
	Cytokines (interleukins)

Cellular events include emigration from blood vessels to site of injury as phagocytosis or killing.

Phagocytosis and killing of Microorganisms

It is the process of taking particulate matter in the cytoplasm by cells.

Pinocytosis

- Taking in fluid particles into the cells
- Discovered by Ellie Metchnikoff in 1884

Steps in phagocytosis

I. Recognition and attachment

Microorganisms are not recognized by neutrophils and macrophages until they are coated by naturally occurring serum proteins.

II. Engulfment regurgitation during feeding

- During degranulation leakage of hydrolytic enzymes, metabolic products ($H_2 O_2$) and lysozymes from neutrophil into outside medium cause tissue damage.
- Kinins released cause vascular dilatation and nerve stimulation.
- Proteases liberated induce tissue damage, platelets aggregate and release PAF4 which is chemotactic to neutrophils and coagulation factors causing polymerization of fibrin.
- PDGF stimulates fibrinogenesis and angiogenesis. Monocytes transform into macrophages to release collagenase, antimicrobial proteases, elastases, complements, IL-1 and TNF. Fever, myalgia and endothelial cell activation.
- Activation of systemic response leads to release of acute phase proteins (complement, fibrinogen, etc.) from the liver and leucocytes and increased haematopoiesis in bone marrow and lymphopoiesis in lymph node and spleen.

III. Killing and Degradation

1) Brought about by reactive oxygen species like hydrogen peroxide (H_2O_2)
2) Myeloperoxidase enzyme present in lysosome of neutrophils
   $H_2O_2 \rightarrow$ HOCl (hypochlorous radical)

   ↓

   Active antimicrobial (kills bacteria)
3) Myeloperoxidase deficient neutrophils

   - superoxide, hydroxyl radicals $\rightarrow H_2O_2$

Terminology of Inflammation

Time	Extent	Exudate	Position	Anatomy	Suffix
Acute	Local	Serous	Parenchymatous	Nephr -	- itis
Chronic	Diffuses	Fibrinous	interstitial	Hepat-	- itis
		Catarrhal		Rhin-	-itis
		Suppurative		Periton-	-itis
		Haemorrhagic		Enter-	-tis
Combination of exudates					

- Sero – fibrinous
- Muco – purulent
- Fibrino – purulent

Fate of Acute Inflammation

- Complete resolution
- Healing by scar formation
- Abscess formation
- Progress to chronic inflammation

Salient steps in acute inflammation

Initiation		
Tissue injury or infection		
• Histamine • Cytokines • Chemokines • PAF • Prostaglandins • Leukotrienes • Bradykinin • C3a / C5a		• Pathogen associated molecular patterns (PAMP) • Pattern recognition receptors
Activation		
Microvasculature		
Blood flow		
Vasodilation		
Activation of endothelium		Activation of neutrophils
Inflammatory mediators	Adhesion molecules	Inflammatory mediators
Outcome		
Slowing / stasis of blood flow		Leukocyte adhesion cascade
Vascular permeability		Leukocyte transmigration across vessel wall
		Chemotaxis
Tissue edema		• **Phagocytosis** • **Microbial killing** • **NET formation** • **Cell debris**
• Opsonization		
• Activation of complement		
• Inactivation of microbes Complement		
• C3a / C5a		
• Membrane attack complex		
• Opsonization		
• Kinins		
• Bradykinin		
Fibrinogen		
• Fibrin meshwork		
• Immobilization of microbes		
• Meshwork for neutrophil migration		
• Fibrinolysis		

NET, Neutrophil extracellular trap, PAF, platelet – activating factor Courtesy: Dr. J.F. Zachary

Killing of Bacteria by neutrophils

↓

Degradation of bacteria by acid hydrolases in granules of neutrophils

↓

TB bacilli aroid degradation by enzymes and present inside phagocytic vacuoles

↓

Spreads infection to other sites through lymphatics

↓

Tissue injury

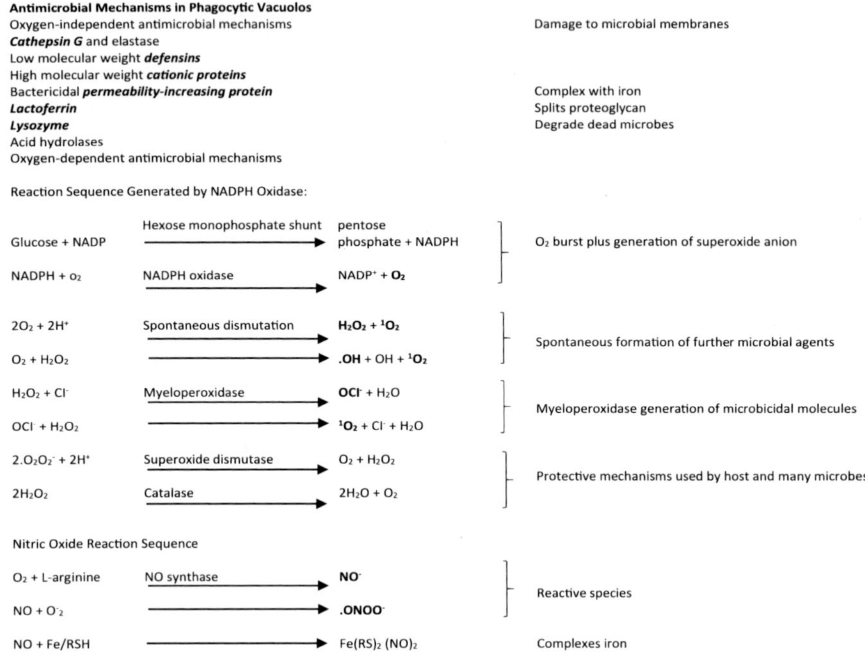

Antimicrobial Mechanisms in Phagocytic Vacuolos

Mechanism			Effect
Oxygen-independent antimicrobial mechanisms			Damage to microbial membranes
Cathepsin G and elastase			
Low molecular weight ***defensins***			
High molecular weight ***cationic proteins***			
Bactericidal ***permeability-increasing protein***			Complex with iron
Lactoferrin			Splits proteoglycan
Lysozyme			Degrade dead microbes
Acid hydrolases			
Oxygen-dependent antimicrobial mechanisms			

Reaction Sequence Generated by NADPH Oxidase:

Reactants	Enzyme / process	Products	Effect
Glucose + NADP	Hexose monophosphate shunt →	pentose phosphate + NADPH	O_2 burst plus generation of superoxide anion
NADPH + o_2	NADPH oxidase →	$NADP^+$ + $\mathbf{O_2}$	
$2O_2 + 2H^+$	Spontaneous dismutation →	$\mathbf{H_2O_2 + {}^1O_2}$	Spontaneous formation of further microbial agents
$O_2 + H_2O_2$	→	**.OH** + OH + $\mathbf{{}^1O_2}$	
$H_2O_2 + Cl^-$	Myeloperoxidase →	$\mathbf{OCl^-}$ + H_2O	Myeloperoxidase generation of microbicidal molecules
$OCl^- + H_2O_2$	→	$\mathbf{{}^1O_2}$ + $Cl^- + H_2O$	
$2.O_2O_2^- + 2H^+$	Superoxide dismutase →	$O_2 + H_2O_2$	Protective mechanisms used by host and many microbes
$2H_2O_2$	Catalase →	$2H_2O + O_2$	

Nitric Oxide Reaction Sequence

Reactants	Enzyme / process	Products	Effect
O_2 + L-arginine	NO synthase →	$\mathbf{NO^-}$	Reactive species
$NO + O^-_2$	→	$\mathbf{.ONOO^-}$	
NO + Fe/RSH	→	$Fe(RS)_2\ (NO)_2$	Complexes iron

Microbicidal species in bold letters. Fe/RSH, a complex of iron with a general sulfhydryl molecule: Fe(RS), oxidized Fe/RSH; O2, superoxide anion, 1O2 single activated oxygen; .OH, hydroxyl free radical; NADPH, reduced nicotinamide adenine dinucleotide phosphate; NADP+, oxidized NADPH; H2O2+ hydrogen peroxide; OCI, hypochlorate anion; NO: nitric oxide, peroxynitrite radical. From Goering R, Dockrell H, Roitt I, et al: Mims' medical microbiology ed 4, St Louis 2008, Mosby

Harmful effects of chemotaxis, phagocytosis

Release of products into the extracellular space-damage tissues

1) Lysosomal enzymes
2) Free radicals
3) Arachidonic acid metabolites like prostaglandins

Classification of Acute Inflammation

Based on the type of exudate

1. Catarrhal or Mucous Inflammation
2. Serous Inflammation
3. Fibrinous Inflammation
4. Suppurative Inflammation (Purulent)
5. Haemorrhagic Inflammation
6. Gangrenous Inflammation

1. Catarrhal or Mucous Inflammation

- Exudate - Mucous
- Site - Occurs in cells capable of producing mucin

Causes

- Mild irritants
- Chemicals (formalin, phenol, detergent)
- Food poisons
- Cold air, dust
- Bacterial and viral infections

Gross Appearance

- Clear, transparent, glistening
- Slimy material containing
- Water and mucous

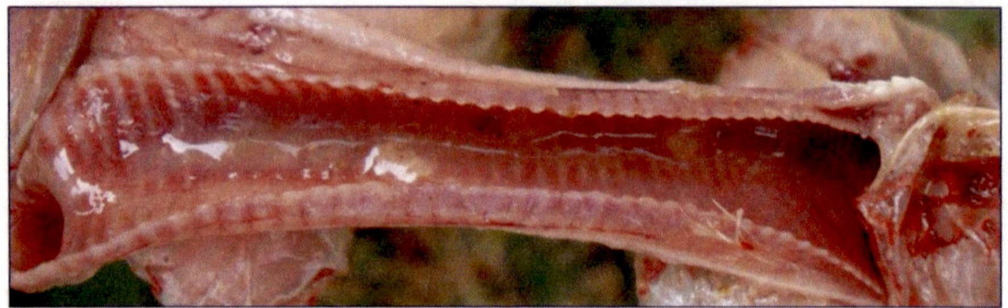

Catarrhal Tracheitis-Broiler Chicken

Microscopical appearance

- Proliferation of epithelial cells
- Desquamation into exudates
- Neutrophils
- Mucus stained blue with haematoxylin

Sequelae

- Recovery if cause is removed
- If not progresses to chronic condition
- On invasion with pyogenic organisms, it becomes mucopurulent
- Fibrosis

2. Serous Inflammation

- Exudate - Plasma or thin watery fluid
- Site - Serous membranes - Peritoneum, pleura, pericardium, joints

Causes

Moderate - severe irritants

- Chemical irritants applied on skin → "BLISTERS"
- Traumatic injury
- Burns
- Viral infections – FMD, vesicular stomatitis

Gross appearance

- Blister formation
- Clear, thin or watery fluid
- Sometimes mixed with fibrin gives a frosty glass appearance

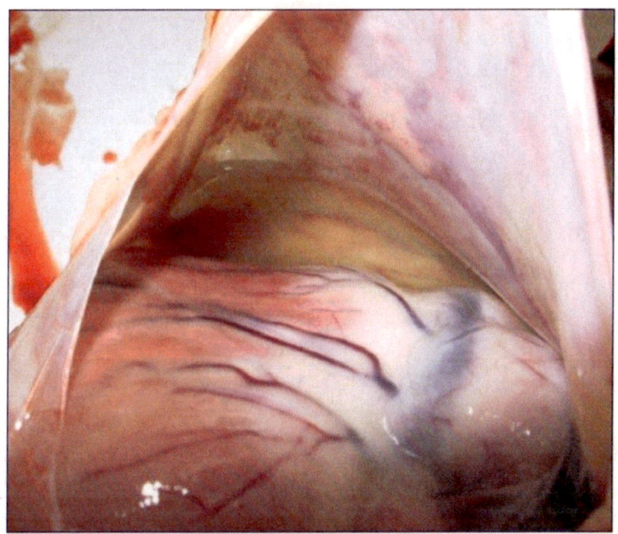

Pericardial sac-Serous exudate

Microscopically

- Homogenous or finely granular exudates
- Stains pink with eosin (intensity varies with amount of protein in the exudates)

Sequelae

- Fluid is resorbed if cause is removed

If not organized or fibrosed, adhesions with cavities will develop with increased in fibrin content

3. Fibrinous Inflammation

- Exudate – Fibrin

Sites

- Body cavities – Pleura, pericardial sac, peritoneum
- Epithelial surfaces (mucous, serous, cutaneous)
- Visceral organs (Lung, liver, kidneys)

Causes – Severe irritant

- Viral diseases - Feline enteritis, malignant catarrhal fever
- Bacterial diseases – Salmonellosis, diphtheria

Gross appearance

- Organ are tenser or hard

Fibrin – stringy, yellowish net–like material

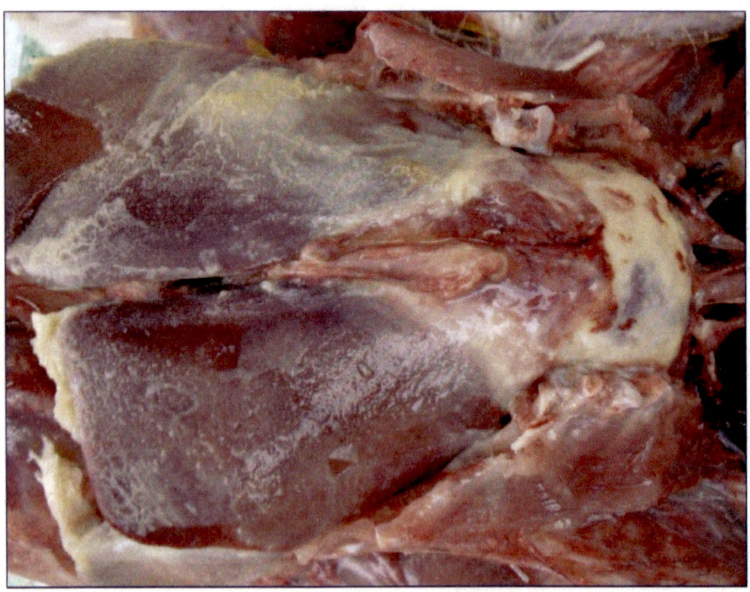

Fibrinous Inflammation –Fowl Liver (*Escherichia coli* infection) -Fibrin covering the hepatic surface (Perihepatitis)

On mucosal surfaces Casts – tubular organs

Pseudomembrane formation

Masses of fibrin not firmly attached to the mucous membrane or peeled off easily.

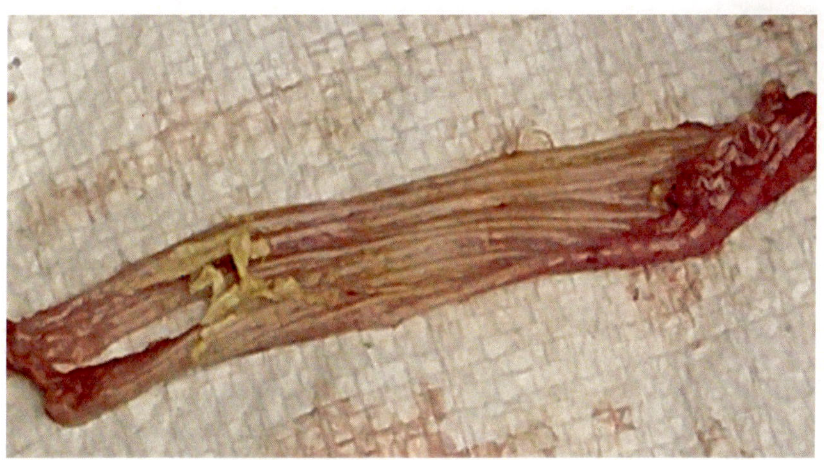

Pseudomembrane-Duck-Oesophagus-Peeled off easily; Not adhered to mucosa

Diphtheretic membrane

Fibrin is firmly attached to the underlying tissue; the tissue undergoes coagulation necrosis

Examples

Diphtheria, swine fever

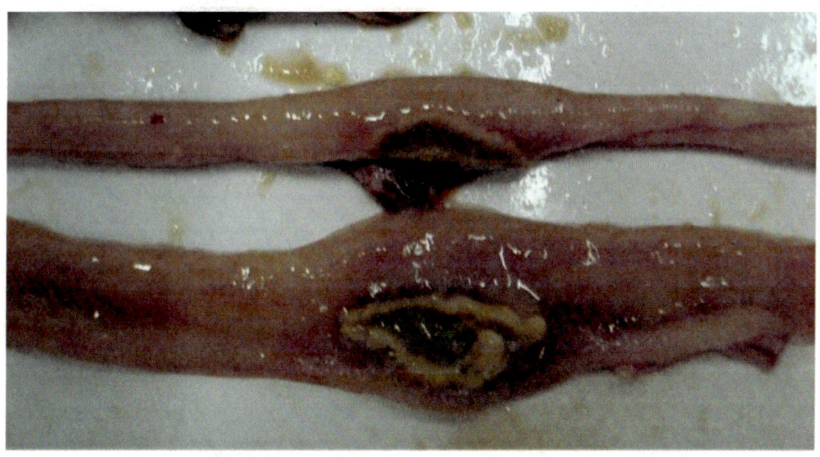

Diphtheritic Inflammation – Chicken- Intestine (Newcastle disease)

True Membrane-Button ulcers

Dead cells are included in exudates.

False Membrane

Without dead epithelial cells "**Bread Butter Appearance**" Fibrinous pericarditis

Microscopical Appearance

- Fibrin appears as dirty pink, net–like
- Entrapment of leucocytes and denuded cells found in the network

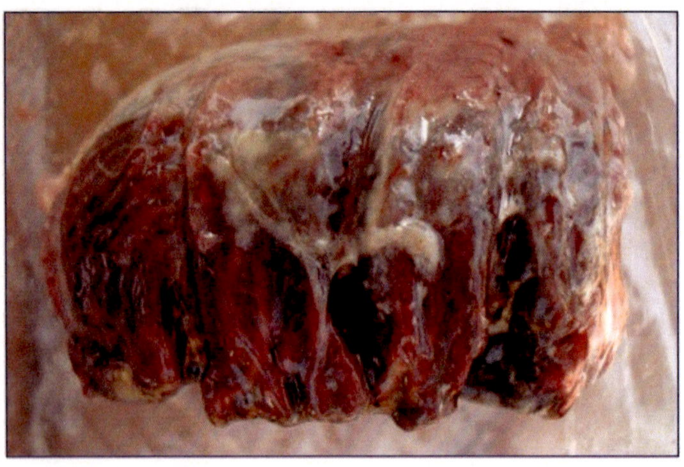

Fibrinous pleuritis-Chicken

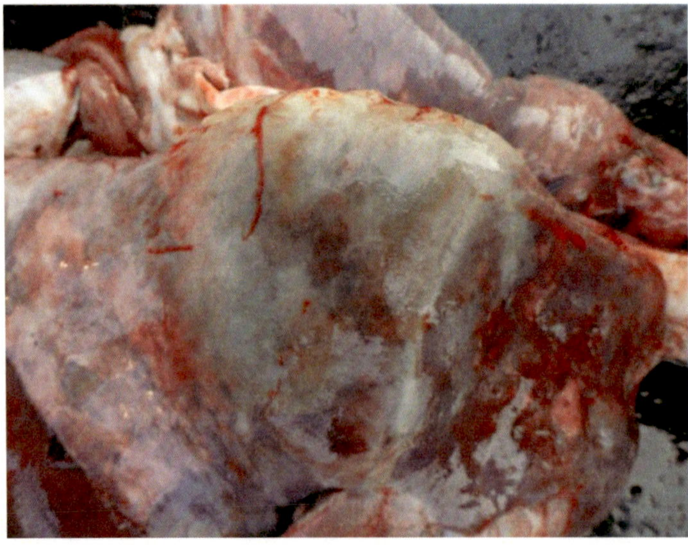

Sheep lung-Pasteurellosis-Serofibrinous pleuropneumonia

Sequelae

Indicates severe injury-Leakage of large fibrinous molecule from blood vessels

Not favorable – Death supervenes. Desquamation of fibrin on epithelial surface Reabsorption from body cavities. Organization

4. Suppurative Inflammation (Purulent)

- Exudate – Pus

Factors Essential for Pus Formation

1. Necrosis
2. Neutrophils
3. Digestion of necrotic tissue by proteolytic enzymes

Causes

Pyogenic bacteria – Staphylococci, Streptococci, *Escherichia coli*

Cornybacterium pyogenes, *Actinomyces bovis* etc

Chemicals – Turpentine, $ZnCl_2$, Mercuric chloride

Suppuration / pus formation is not commonly seen in rabbits

- Due to the presence of antienzyme against proteases
- Tuberculosis

Characteristics of pus

i. Necrotic tissue/cells
ii. Serum Alkaline – P^H
iii. Color – white, yellow, green, red or black, red
iv. Consistency – thin, watery or creamy, thick
v. Pus serum – liquor puris - does not coagulate

Types of Suppurative Inflammatory Conditions

Cellulitis - Diffuse spreading suppurative inflammation of connective tissue

Abscess - Collection of pus locally within a closed cavity in an organ or tissue

Pyogenic Membrance

- Limiting wall formed by partly damaged and partly living - where active warfare is going on to limit the spread of infection.

Ulcer

- The discontinuity of skin or mucous membrane – resulting in opening of abscess

Sinus - Tract in the tissues communicating with an epithelial surface discharging pus from an abscess

Fistula -Tract connects two epithelial surfaces such as skin and mucous membrane to discharge pus from an abscess

Boil / Furuncle - Small suppurative inflammation on skin which involves hair follicle or sebaceous gland – caused by *Staphyloccos aureus*

Pustule - Circumscribed cavity in the epidermis with pus

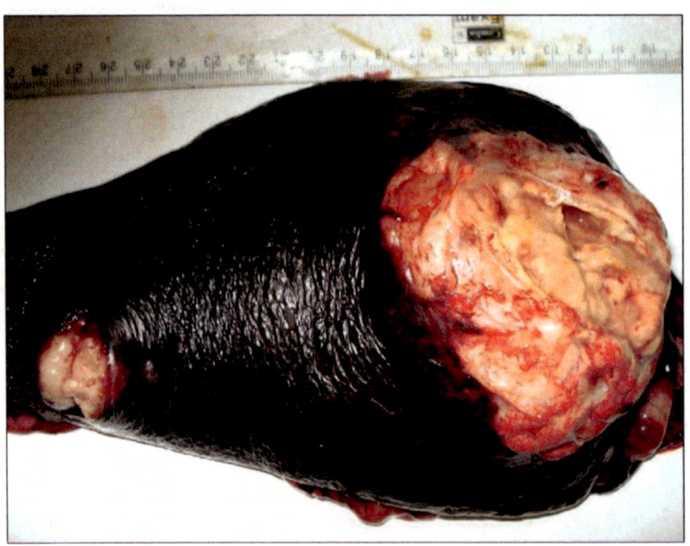

Suppurative Inflammation -Splenic Abscess -Dog

5. Haemorrhagic Inflammation

Exudate - Blood

Cause - violent / severe irritant causes damage to blood vessels, Bacterial diseases– Black quarter, anthrax, haemorrhagic septicaemia

Viral – Infectious laryngotracheitis in poultry

Protozoal – Intestinal coccidiosis in poultry

Gross - Presence of blood

Microscopical - RBC's in exudate

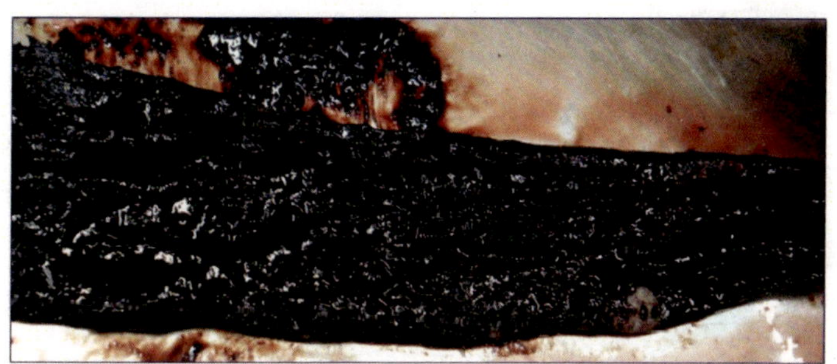

Haemorrhagic inflammation - Tarry/black coloured digested blood -Intestine-Dog

6. Gangrenous Inflammation

Necrotic tissue is invaded by saprophytic (live on dead tissues) organisms causing gangrene

Thrombosis of blood vessels - ischaemia

↓

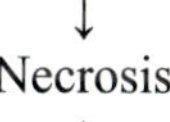

Necrosis

↓

Invaded by saprophytes e.g. – Black Quarter (*Clostridium chauvoei*)

↓

Gangrene (Green in colour; foul smelling (H_2S,FeS)

Chemical Mediators of Inflammation

Chemical mediators are found

I. Cells

i. **Preformed-** Vasoactive amines e.g., Histamine, serotonin and lysosomal enzymes

ii. **Newly Synthesized-** Prostaglandins, Leukotrienes, Platelet Activating Factor-PAF, Cytokines

II. Plasma complement system, kinin system, clotting, fibrinolysin system

I. Cellular

i. Preformed mediator in secretory granules

Mediators	Sources
Histamine	Mast cell, basophils, platelets
Serotonin	Platelets
Lysosomal enzymes	Neutrophils

ii. Newly synthesised mediators and its source

Mediators	Sources
Prostaglandin	All leukocytes, platelets, Endothelial cell
Leukotrienes	All leucocytes
Platelet activating factor	All leucocytes, endothelial cell
Activated oxygen species	All leucocytes
Nitric oxide	Macrophages
Cytokines	Lymphocytes, macrophages

II. Plasma-Liver

a. Factor XII (Hageman factor) activation – kinin system (Bradykinin), Coagulation system

b. Complement activation – C3a, C5a – Anaphylatoxins, C3b – phagocytosis of bacteria, C5b-9 – Membrane attack complex (MAC)

Biologic activity

a. Specific receptors on target cells

b. Direct-enzymes

c. Mediate oxidative damage

Chemical Mediators

- Stimulate release and mediation of target cells themselves.
- The secondary mediators have similar or opposite effect.
- Chemical action – one or many target cells with different effects.
- Chemical mediators are short lived and scavenge oxygen species.
- Histamine and serotonin cause tissue damage.

i. Preformed Mediators in Secretory Granules

Histamine

- Histamine is found in the granules of mast cells, basophils and platelets. It increases the vascular permeability of venules and dilates arterioles and induces endothelial junctional gap early response to inflammation.

Serotonin

- **Serotonin (5-hydroxy tryptamine) -** It is present in mast cell and platelets of rodents. It increases vascular permeability and involved in early inflammatory response

Lysosomal components

- Lysosomal components leak during phagocytosis or regurgitation.

  Small granules contain lysosomes, collagen, alkaline phosphatase, histaminases and plasminogen activator. Large granules (azurophils) contain myeloperoxidases, bactericidal factor, acid hydrolases and neutral proteases which are responsible for vascular permeability, chemotaxis and tissue damage.

Lysozyme

- Lysozyme (neuraminidase) is found in granulocytes, monocytes and macrophages and produced by epithelial cells of mucosa and glands of intestinal tract and secreted in milk, tear and saliva. Lysozyme catalyses the hydrolysis of peptidoglycans in bacterial cell wall.

ii. Newly synthesised mediators and its sources

Arachidonic acid metabolites

- The cell membrane phospholipids of neutrophils are acted upon by phospholipases.
- When arachidonic acid enters 5-lipoxygenase pathway, leukotrienes (LT) are produced e.g. LTc4, LTD4, LTE4.
- When acted through platelets lipoxins which are potent chemoattractants are produced.
- If acted by cyclooxgenase pathway, prostaglandins (PG) are produced.

Eicosanoids

- These are derived from arachidonic acid from injured cell membrane phospholipids.
- These are prostaglandins and leukotrienes. Prostaglandin derivatives PGI2, PGE2, PGD2 cause vasodilatation while thromboxaneA2, LTC4, LTD4, LTE4 cause vasoconstriction.
- LTC4, LTD4, LTE4 are also responsible for increased vascular permeability. LTD4 and HETE can induce chemotaxis and leucocytic adhesion

Arachidonic Acid Metabolites

(Prostaglandins, Leukotrienes, Lipoxins)

Formation and action of mediators are given.

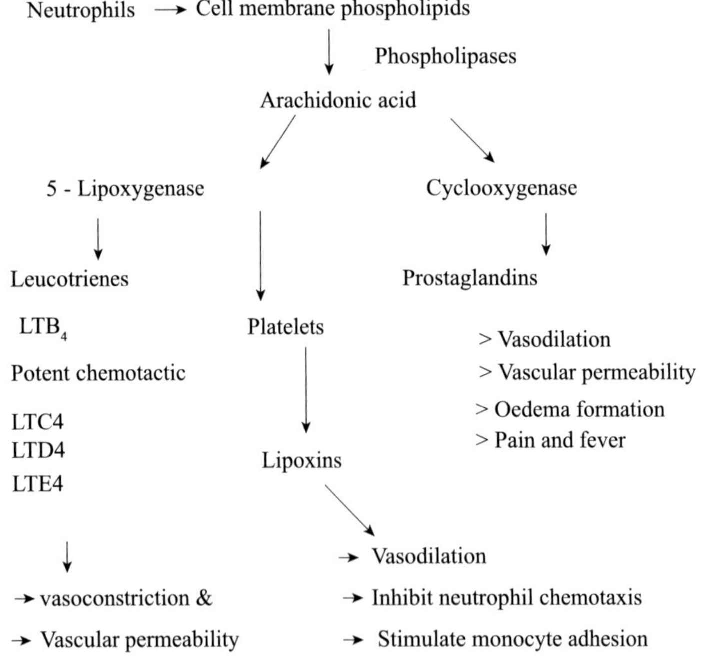

Leukotrienes are 1000 times more potent than histamine. II. Plasma Protein System

Plasma proteases

(Kinin, Clotting, Fibrinolytic systems)

Now let us see the formation and action of plasma proteases

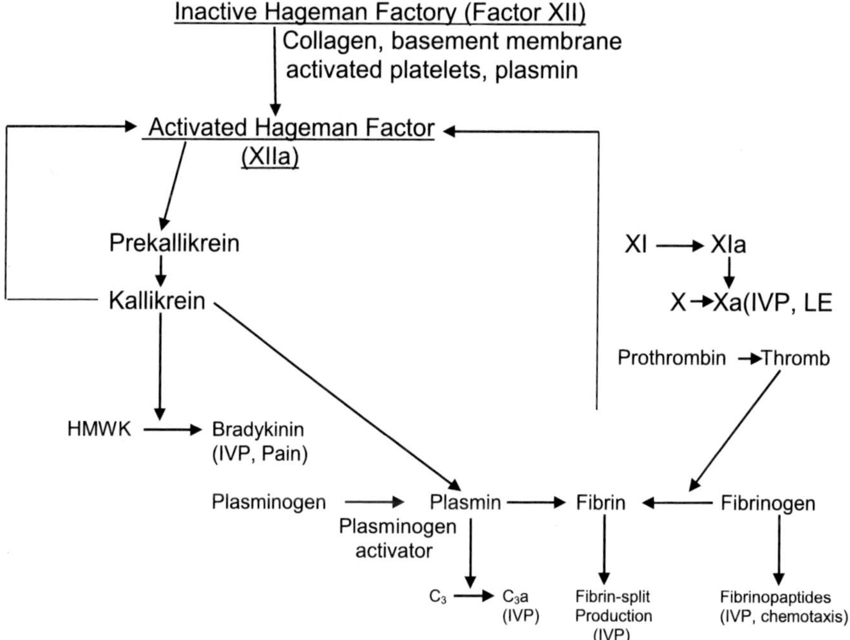

i. Kinin, clotting and fibrinolytic system

Kinin system

- The Hageman factor (factor XII) is activated on contact with collagen, basement membrane and platelets to produce prekallikrein.
- The prekallikrein is converted to kallikrein which will be converted to bradykinin that induces vascular permeability, pain and smooth muscle contraction.
- Kallikrein also mediates plasminogen, vascular permeability and vascular dilatation.
- Activated Hageman factor is also involved in conversion of prothrombin to thrombin which in turn aids in conversion of fibrinogrn to fibrin.
- The fibrinolytic peptides and split products of fibrin can induces vascular

permeability and chemotaxis.

- The vasoactive polypeptide (kinins) are derived from kininogen (plasma globulins).
- The kinins are potent mediator of vasodilatation, pain, increased capillary permeability.
- The bradykinin induces vascular leakage from post capillary venules. It is 10 times more active than histamine but short lived.

Interrelationships between the four-plasma mediator system triggered by activation of factor XII (Hageman factor)

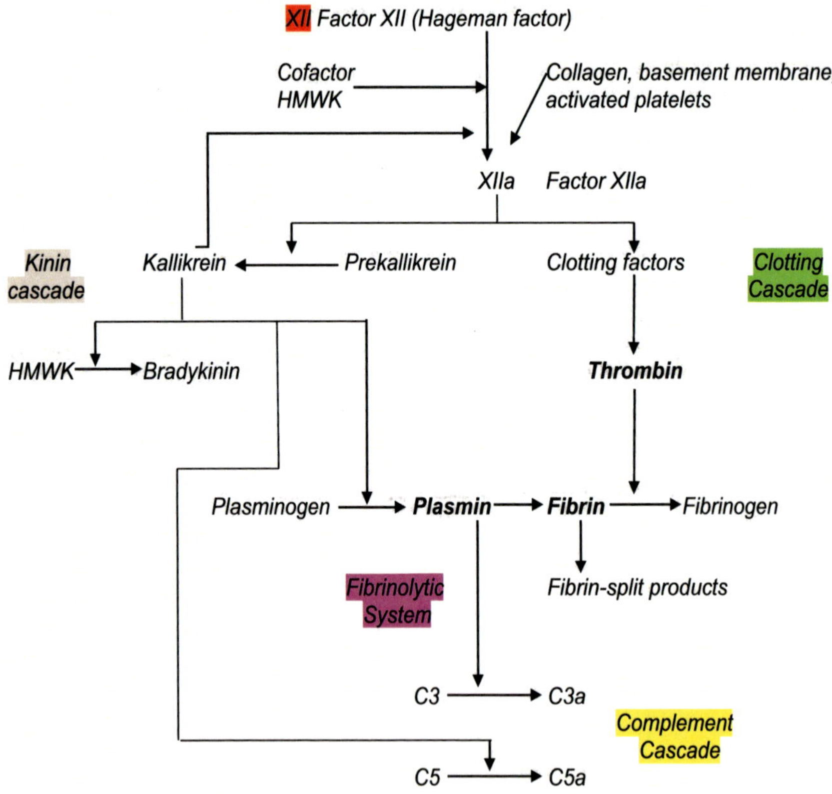

Complement system

- Complement, represented as C, consists of 20 proteins in an inactive form in plasma and body fluids.
- Complement is mainly synthesised by liver. Complement system may be activated in one of the two ways, classic or alternate pathway.

- But both the pathways converge to produce a membrane attack complex (MAC) which is responsible for lysis of bacterial cell membrane and also results in mediating inflammation. e.g. chemotaxis, histamine release from mast cells (C3a) and procoagulant from platelets.
- C3b is a major opsonin protein which adhere to bacteria (opsonisation). It is recognised, phagocytosed and destroyed by neutrophils and monocytes.

Complement activation Mechanisms

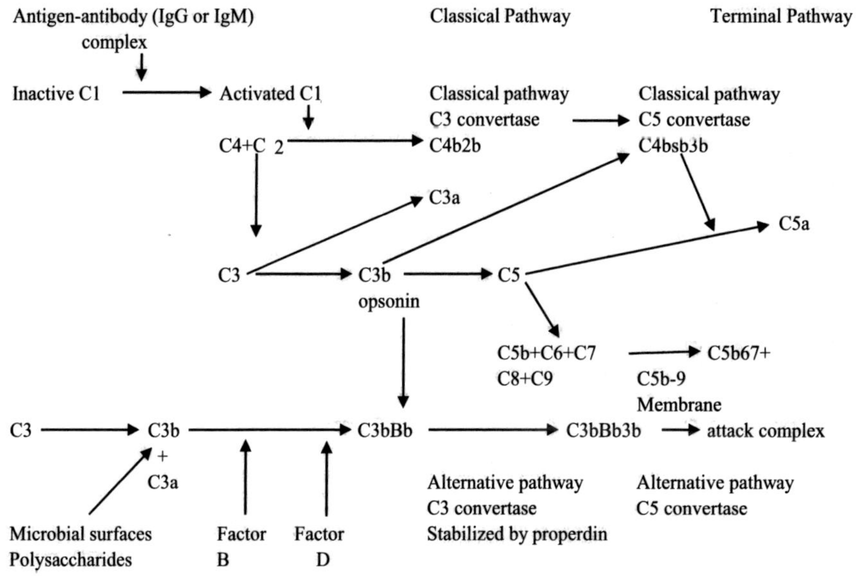

Alternative Pathway

The Main Functions of Complement

Activities	Associated Complement Protein
Host Defense	
Opsonization	C3 and C4 fragments
Chemotaxis and leukocyte activation	C5a, C3a, C4a, and leukocyte receptors
Lysis of microbial cell walls	Membrane attack complex(C5b-C9)
Bridging Innate and Adaptive Immunity	
Augmentation of antibody response	C3b, C4b immune complexes and antigen; C3 receptors on B lymphocytes and antigen presenting cells
Enhancement of immunologic memory	C3b, C4b immune complexes and antigen; C3 receptors on follicular dendritic cells

Disposal Of Waste	
Clearance of immune complexes	C1q; C3 and C4 fragments
Clearance of apoptotic cells	C1q; C3 and C4 fragments

ii. Clotting (antifibrinolytic) system

Coagulation is seen following damage of endothelium in inflammation through fibrinolytic system, initiated by activated Hageman factor.

Fibrinolytic system

Tissue plasminogen activator (tPA) and urokinase are major activators of fibrinolysis by cleaving plasminogen into plasmin. Fibrinolytic mechanism controls clotting by breaking fibrin thereby solubilizing the fibrin clot. Otherwise, uncontrolled clotting will occur in the whole vascular system.

Antifibrinolytic system

1. Plasminogen activator inhibitor-1 (PAI-1) inhibits these activators to decrease fibrinolysis.
2. Thrombin-activatable fibrinolysis inhibitor (TAFI), which inhibits binding of plasminogen/tPA to fibrin, and
3. Antiplasmin, which bind to and inhibit activity of plasmin that has disassociated from the fibrin-platelet aggregate.

Actions of Mediators in Acute Inflammation

Action	Mediators
Vasodilation	Histamine Prostaglandins Nitric oxide
Vascular permeability	Vasoactive amines C3a and C5a Bradykinin Leukotrienes C4, d4, E4 Platelet activating factor Substance P
Leukocyte chemotaxis and activation	C5a Leukotriene B4 Chemokines TNF and IL-1
Fever	TNF and IL-1 prostaglandins
Pain	Prostaglandins Bradykinin

Salient Mechanism of Acute Inflammation

Primary Mediators of the Process

Vasodilation

Nitric oxide

Bradykinin

Prostaglandins: PGD2

Leukotrienes: LTB4

LPS activation

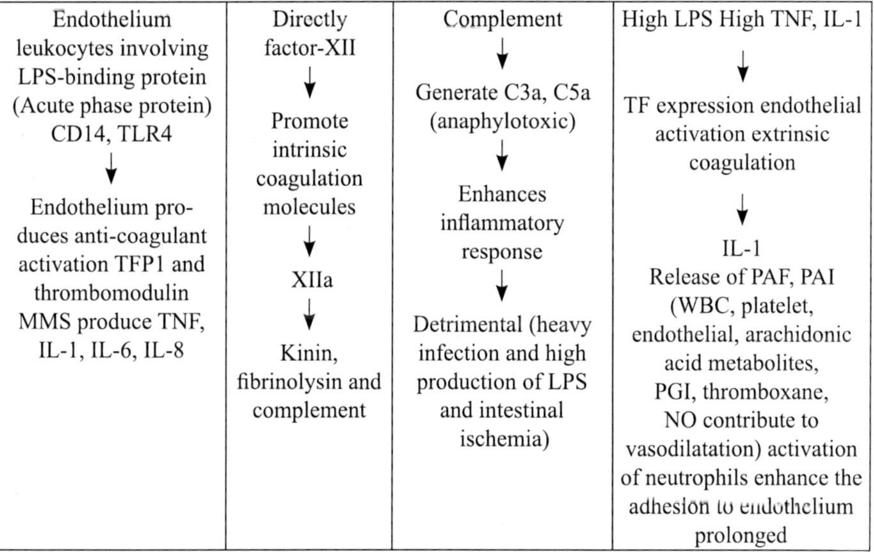

Endothelium leukocytes involving LPS-binding protein (Acute phase protein) CD14, TLR4 ↓ Endothelium produces anti-coagulant activation TFP1 and thrombomodulin MMS produce TNF, IL-1, IL-6, IL-8	Directly factor-XII ↓ Promote intrinsic coagulation molecules ↓ XIIa ↓ Kinin, fibrinolysin and complement	Complement ↓ Generate C3a, C5a (anaphylotoxic) ↓ Enhances inflammatory response ↓ Detrimental (heavy infection and high production of LPS and intestinal ischemia)	High LPS High TNF, IL-1 ↓ TF expression endothelial activation extrinsic coagulation ↓ IL-1 Release of PAF, PAI (WBC, platelet, endothelial, arachidonic acid metabolites, PGI, thromboxane, NO contribute to vasodilatation) activation of neutrophils enhance the adhesion to endothelium prolonged

Increased Vascular Permeability

Vasoactive amines: histamine, substance P, bradykinin

Complement factors: C5a, C3a

Fibrinopeptides and fibrin breakdown products

Prostaglandins: PGE_2

Leukotrienes: LTB, LTC, LTD4, LTE4

PAF, substance P Cytokines: IL-1, TNF

Smooth Muscle Contraction

Histamine Serotonin C3a Bradykinin PAF

Leukotriene D4

Chemotaxis, Leukocyte Activation

Complement factors: C5a

Leukotrienes: LTB4

Chemokines: IL-8

Defensins: a- and ß-Defensins

Bacterial products: LPS, peptidoglycan, teichoic acid

Collagenous lectins: Ficolins, surfactant proteins A and D, mannan-binding lectin

Cytokines: IL-1, TNF Surfactant proteins A and Da

Fever

Cytokines: IL-1, TNF, IL-6, Prostaglandins: PGE2

Nausea

Cytokines: IL-1, TNF, high mobility group factors

Pain Bradykinin Prostaglandins: PGE2

Tissue Damage

Caused by neutrophil and macrophage lysosomal/granule contents: Matrix metalloproteinases

Reactive oxygen species: Superoxide anion, hydroxyl radical, nitric oxide

Chronic Inflammation

Characteristics

- Infiltration with mononuclear cells
- Tissue destruction and repair
- New blood vessel formation (angiogenesis) and fibrosis
- Long duration

- Follow acute inflammation – persistence of causative agent
- Chronic from the beginning – irritants of low intensity

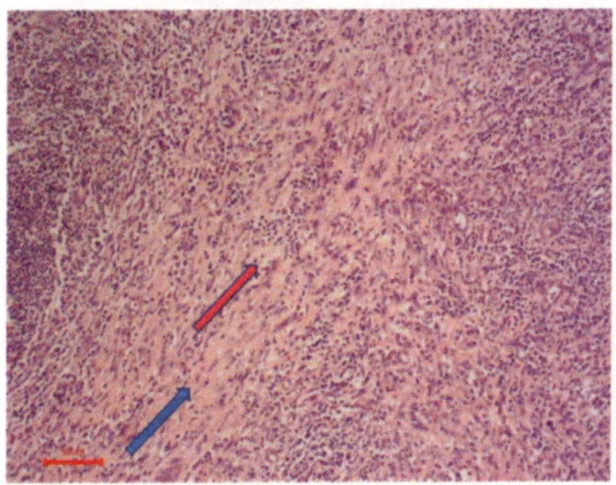

Chronic inflammation-Fibrous tissue (Blue arrow); blood vessel (Red arrow)

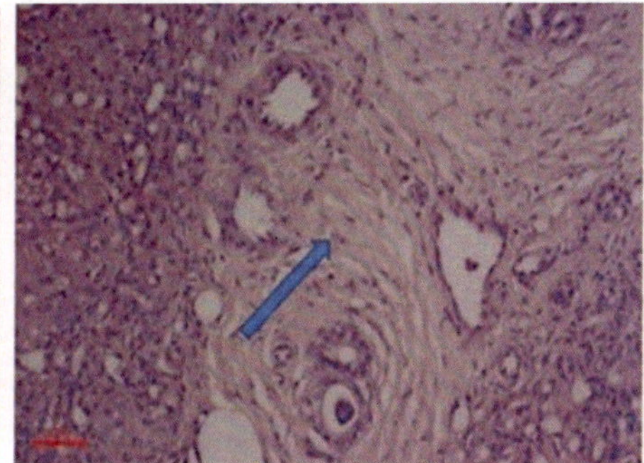

Chronic Inflammation-Liver-Portal fibrosis (Arrow)

e,g. – Tuberculosis, Johne's disease, Fungal diseases

- Prolonged exposure to toxic agents

e.g. – Asbestos, silica particles

Causes of Chronic Inflammation

- Bacteria – *Pasteurella aviseptica*, *Erysipelothrix rhusiopathiae*
- Phytotoxins – Crotalaria, senecio
- Foreign bodies – sharp objects, dust, worms, inert objects
- • Constant and repeated mechanical irritation
- e.g.: kennel granuloma, calluses

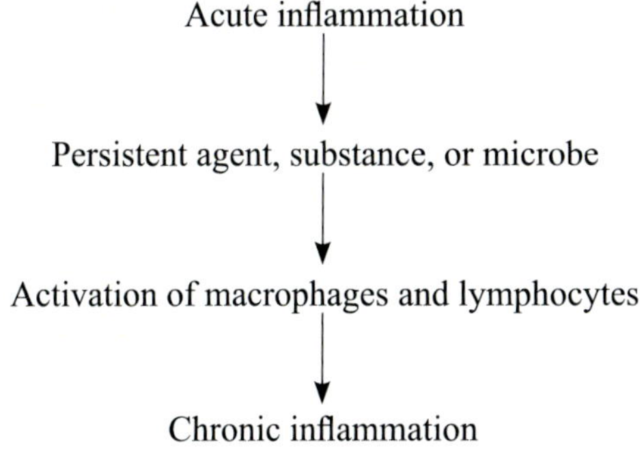

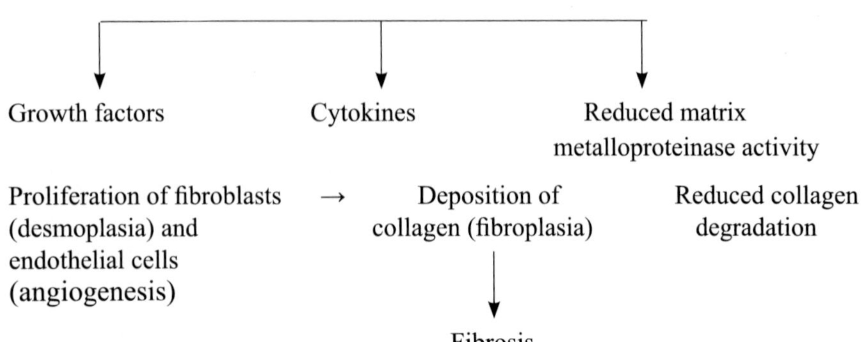

Cytokines

- These are derived from activated macrophages and lymphocytes and are proteins e.g. TNFα, IL-1 are produced by macrophages.
- γ-Interferon also induces acute phase response whereas interleukin 10 is a potent anti inflammatory cytokine.

Platelet activating factor (PAF)

- PAF is derived from degeneration of membrane phospholipids (platelets, neutrophils, endothelium).
- PAF causes increased vascular permeability and 100 to 10,000 times more potent than histamine.
- Higher concentration of platelet activating factor can stimulate platelets, enhance leucocyte adhesion to endothelium and stimulate vasoconstriction..

IL-2 and TNF can produce endothelial activation adhesion of leucocytes production of arachidonic acid metabolite and nitric oxide.

Chemokines

- Chemokines are responsible for activation and migration of leucocytes in acute inflammation.
- alpha chemokines (C-H-C)- attract neutrophils, beta chemokines (C-C) attract monocytes, lymphocytes, eosinophils and basophils, gamma chemokines (C) attracts lymphocytes and CX3C causes attraction and adhesion of monocytes and T-cells.

- Acute phase proteins - They are not normally present in plasma but markedly increased after injury.
- Hence, it is of diagnostic value in inflammation.
- Chemokines are synthesized in liver in response to cytokines released by inflammation leucocytes (IL-1, TNF alpha)

Examples Function of Acute Phase Protein

- Fibrinogen, fibrin coagulation forming coagulant polymers
- C3 Backbone of complement cascade responsible for destruction of bacteria
- C-reactive protein: Initiating complement dependent opsonisation
- Haptoglobulin: Antioxidant by binding haemoglobin and saving iron

Interferons

- Interferons are produced by host cells in response to stimulation by virus, intracellular bacteria, foreign material and soluble protein.
- It is considered as first host defence against viral infection.
- Fibronectin, an alpha 2 glycoprotein on fibroblast surface and basement membrane.
- When in plasma helps in opsonisation of bacteria and promotes phagocytosis.

Oxygen Derived Free Radicals

- Oxygen derived free radicals (superoxide, hydrogen peroxide and hydroxide radicals) derived from membrane damage like neutrophils can cause tissue injury and endothelial damage.

Nitric Oxide

- Nitric oxide (NO) - Microbicidal agent in activated macrophages causes vascular dilatation.
- It is soluble and short lived free radical gas.
- Activation of Hageman factor results in cascade of reactions. The fragment which enhances inflammatory process and this stimulates complement system, kinin system, clotting system and fibrinolytic system.

Macrophage Activation Process

Stimulus I

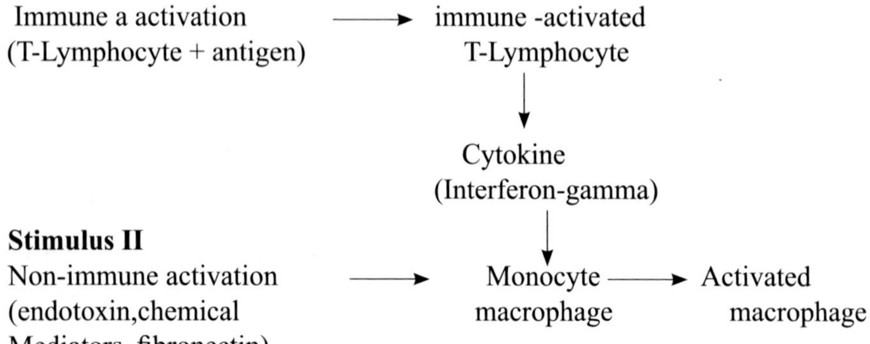

Activated macrophage products cause tissue destruction and fibrosis

Tissue Injury	Fibrosis
Toxic oxygen metabolites	Growth factors (PDGF, FGF, TGF- beta)
Proteases	Fibrogenic cytokines
Neutrophil chemotactic factors	Angiogenesis factors (FGF)
Nitric oxide (NO)	Remodelling' collagenases

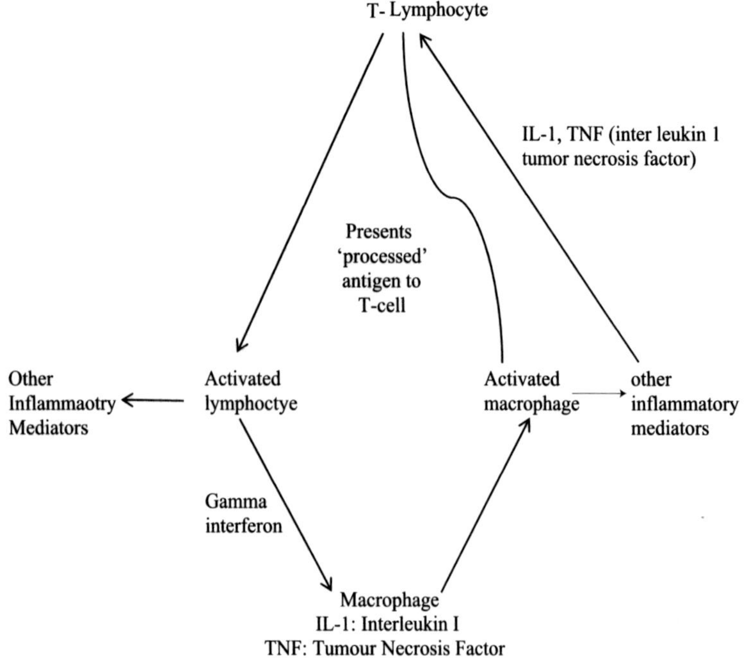

Gross Appearance

- Gray and firm, white, tough, hard (mature variety), nodules (granuloma) kidney – pitted appearance
- Smooth, dense, watery (newly formed)
- Yellowish, soft and easily cut

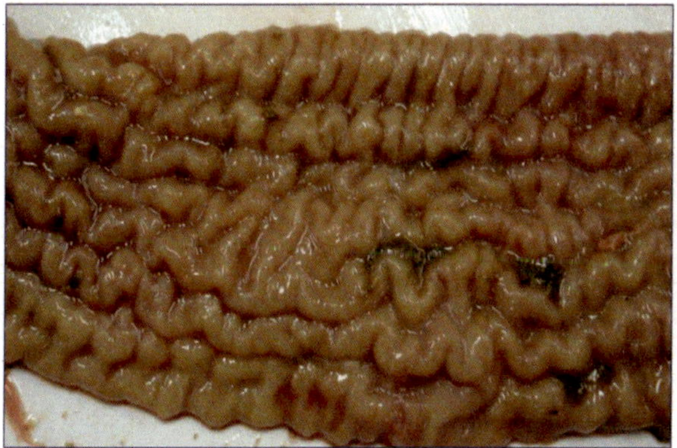

Chronic Inflammation-Cattle- Johne's disease- -Corrugated Intestine

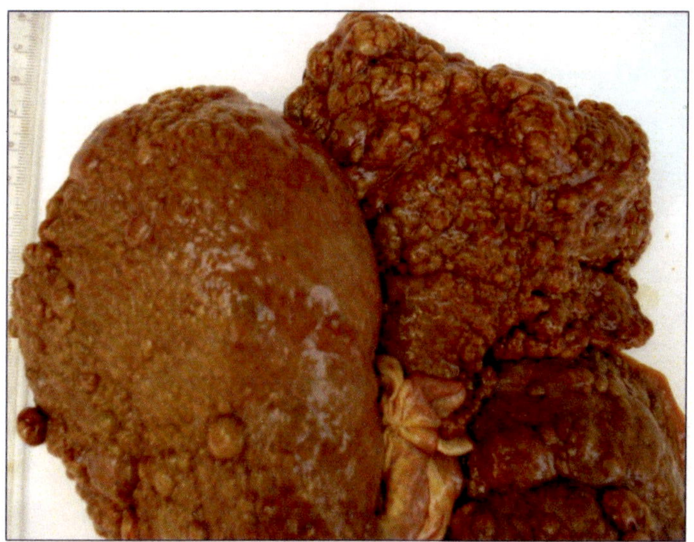

Chronic Inflammation-Liver-Shrunken-Multiple nodular cirrhosis

Microscopical Appearance

- Vascular and cellular response is less
- Proliferation of fibrous connective tissue
- New blood vessel formation
- Mononuclear cells – predominant

  Macrophages

  Plasma cells

  Lymphocytes
- Giant cells
- Neutrophils — in bacterial infection
- Encapsulation

Two types of Chronic Inflammation

1. This may be sequel of persistent and resolved acute inflammation
2. It may develop as a slowly evolving chronic process without an acute inflammatory phase

1. Persistent acute inflammation

- The lesions of persistent inflammation are progressively dominated by the presence of macrophages, fibrous tissue and blood vessels e.g. Acute fibrinous pericarditis - infiltrated with fibroblasts and collagen if not resolved.
- **Chronic active inflammation** includes apart from neutrophils, presence of macrophages and plasma cells which may be associated with osteomyelitis, metritis and epididymitis (Brucellosis).
- These are mostly caused by bacteria and fungi predisposed with deficient immunocompetency.

2. Evolving chronic inflammation

- Diseases like tuberculosis, actinobacillosis and osteoarthritis in which chronic inflammation begins as an asymptomatic process in which neutrophils are not present but infiltrated with macrophages which deals with persistent injury.
- It lacks cardinal signs of acute inflammation.

3. Granulomatous inflammation

- This is a form of chronic inflammatory process in which aggregates of large highly activated macrophages are present.
- When the macrophages take up bacteria, fungi, aberrant parasite (Toxocara larva) or inert substances (silica, asbestos) which cannot be killed or fully digested, monocytes are attracted to the site that are not ineffective in phagocytosis.
- So that the cells continue to infiltrate the lesion and are found in large numbers.
- The macrophages become larger and foamy because of accumulation of causative agents, debris from an injured tissue.
- So this foamy macrophages are referred to as an **epithelioid cells** which are the **hall mark of granulomatous inflammation**.
- The granulomatous lesions develop slowly over a period of several weeks or months before producing clinical signs of disease.
- The microorganisms involved do not cause endothelial damage and are not chemoattractive, so that acute inflammatory signs and neutrophils are not seen.

Other ways of Classification of Chronic Inflammation

1. Chronic inflammation – Simple type, predominantly cellular exudates containing lymphocytes, macrophages and plasma cells are fewer.

Sometimes both lymphocytes and macrophages may predominate (lympho-histiocytic) seen in early stages of chronic inflammation like viral infection.

2. Chronic active inflammation

Besides cellular components of chronic inflammation, it also contains neutrophils, fibrin and plasma protein of acute inflammatory response.

3. Granulomatous inflammation

- **Basic cellular exudate -** Predominantly activated macrophages, also epithelioid macrophages, giant cells and lesser number of lymphocytes and plasma cells. e.g. deep seated mycoses, bacterial infection with Nocardia, Brucella, Mycobacteria and protozoa
  - Chronic inflammation
  - Circumscribed lesion

- No exudates or cellular changes
- The histiocytes (macrophages) in the lesion have large amount of cytoplasm and resemble epithelial cells called "**Epithelioid Cells**"
- Epitheloid cells fuse to form "Giant Cells"
- Foreign body giant cell e.g. **Langhan's cell**

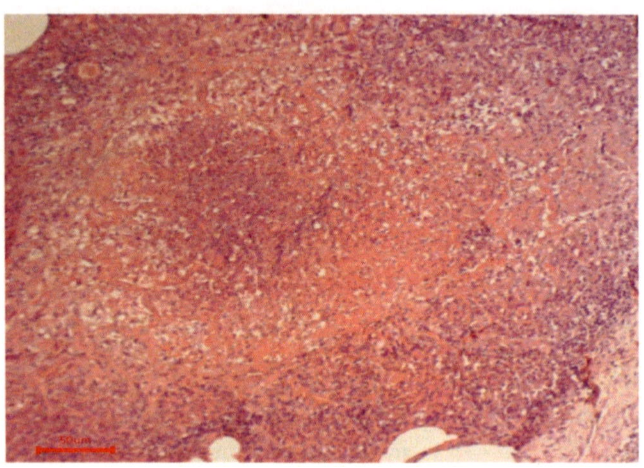

Tuberculous granuloma

Causes for Granulomatous Inflammation

- Bacteria – TB, JD, Actinomycosis, Actinobacillosis
- Fungus – *Aspergillus fumigatus*
- Foreign bodies – Silica, asbestos, inert material

Result

- Helps in localising the infection
- Allows inflammatory and immune mechanism to act for longer periods of time

4. Pyogranulomatous inflammation

- This type of inflammation contains similar cellular exudates like granulomatous inflammation that multifocal infiltration of neutrophils, fibrin and plasma proteins.
- A nodule like granulomatous areas with neutrophils is termed as pyogranuloma e.g. Common in blastomycosis.

5. Granuloma

- Distinct type with well defined macrophage infiltration. Usually it can be non-caseating or caseating.
- Non-caseating granulomas are round to oval containing numerous macrophages, variable epithelioid macrophages, some multinucleated giant cells, peripheral zone of fibroblast, lymphocyte and plasma cells.
- In caseating granuloma, the centre is having grey-white, yellow pasty necrotic debris resembling cheese (Latin caseous = cheese) e.g. tuberculosis

Granuloma

Foreign body granuloma	Immune mediated granuloma
Relatively inert foreign body (talc, i/v drug abuse, suture materials Other fibre large enough to preclude phagocytosis by a single macrophage Do not incite inflammation or an immune response Epithelioid cells and Giant cells seen Foreign body at the centre (polarized light refractile) Granuloma forms but is not static	Insoluble material Capable of inducing cell mediated immunity (CMI) CMI need not form granuloma But when insoluble or particulate **Granuloma if forms,** pathogenesis Macrophage engulf and process the substance Present to T-lymphocyte Gets activated to produce IL – 2 Which activate other T-cells with perpetuation IFN – gamma produced transform (important steps) macrophage to epithelioid cells

Result of Chronic Inflammation

- Delayed healing
- Permanent change or scar formation
- Distortion / Disfigurement of the organ / tissue (Inflammatory cells displace, replace or obliterate the tissue)
- Impairs mobility
- Epithelial surface – hyperplasia – Metaplasia – Neoplasia
- Increase intracranial pressure - destruction neurons and glia

Differences Between Acute and Chronic Inflammation

Acute	Chronic
Short duration	Long duration
Irritant – Severe	Low intensity
Marked vascular changes	Less prominent vascular changes
Profuse exudate	Scanty
Soft in consistency	Hard in consistency
No fibrosis	Proliferation of fibrovascular connective tissue and epithelium

Allergic Inflammation

Animal / person previously sensitized to foreign bodies

Diagnosis of JD, TB, Glanders

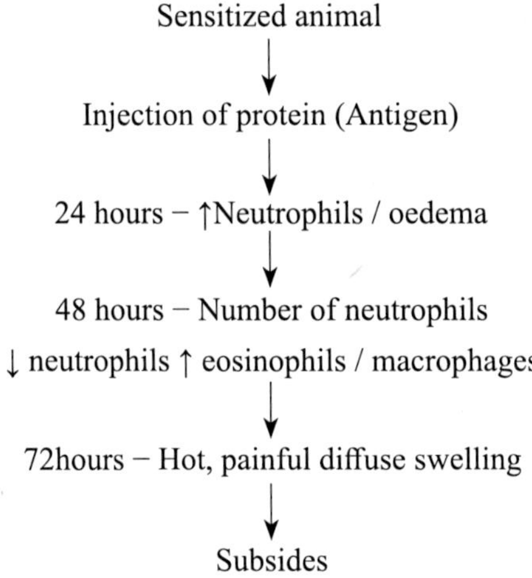

Viral Inflammation

- Obligatory parasites
- Cannot survive outside the cells
- Once inside the cell, protected against antibodies
- **"INCLUSION BODIES"** – aggregates of virus Basophilic – replication is complete Acidophilic – ongoing replication

  Intracytoplasmic – i/c – Fowl pox, vaccinia, rabies

  Intranuclear – i/n – infectious canine hepatitis

  i/c and i/n – Small pox, Canine distemper

- **Reactions of cells to virus**
- Hyperplasia – Shope papilloma virus
- Hyperplasia and necrosis – Fowl pox

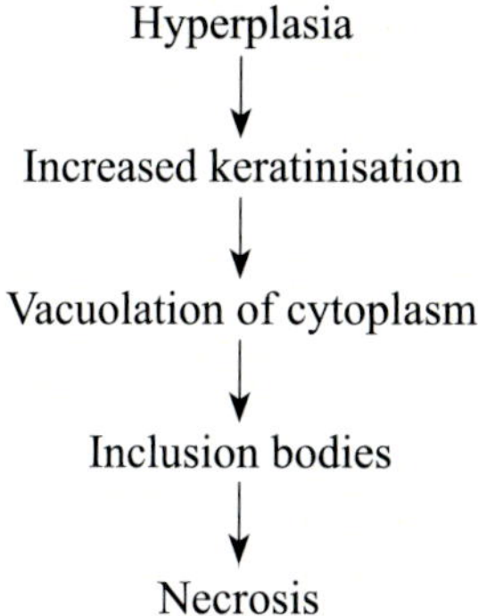

Proliferation quickly followed by necrosis e.g.

Vaccinia; Necrosis alone – FMD; Rabies – Cytocidal Inflammatory cells -

Lymphocytes, plasma cells, macrophages

No neutrophils

No suppuration

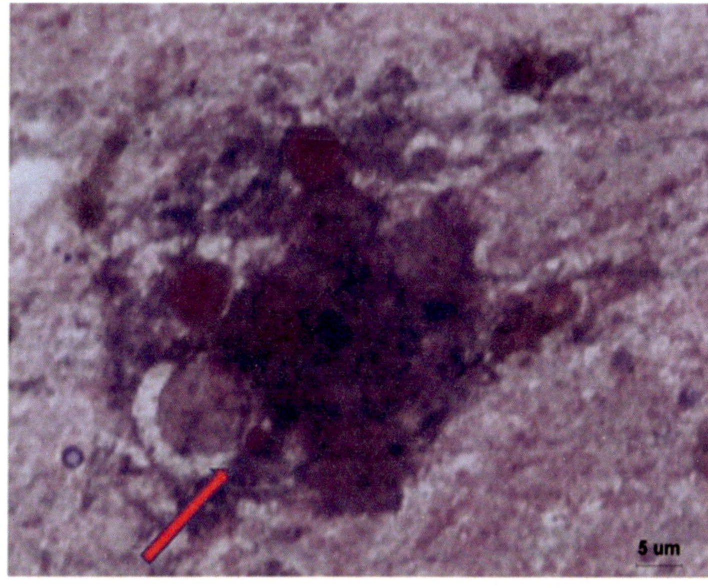

Eosinophilic intracytoplasmic inclusion bodies (Red arrow)-Rabies

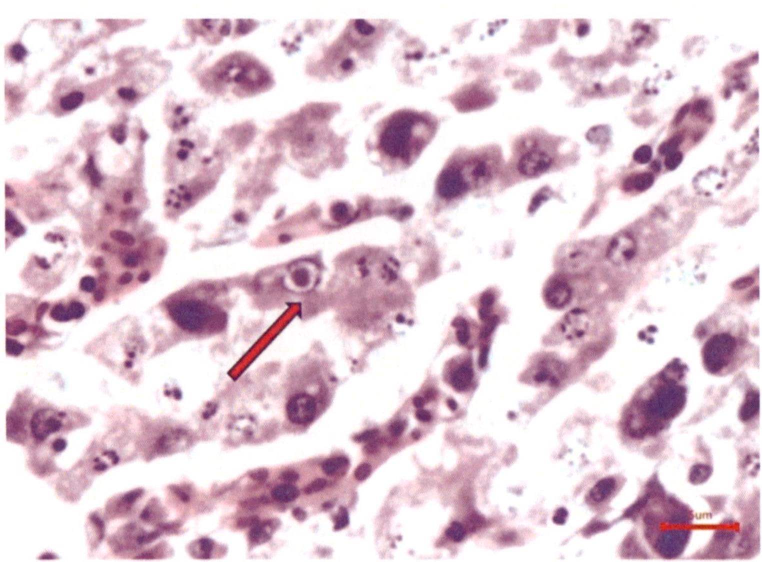

Eosinophilic intraneclear inclusion bodies (Red-arrow) – Fowl-Inclusion body hepatitis

Rickettsial Inflammation

- *Anaplasma marginale, Ehrlichia canis, Chlamydia psittaci*
- They are all bacteria
- Obligatory parasites
- Transmitted through arthropod vectors

Cells in Inflammatory Response

Neutrophils

Synonyms etc.

- Granulocytes
- Microphages of Metchnikoff
- Polymorphonuclear cells (PMN cells)
- First line of cellular defense
- Pus cells
- Heterophils-chicken, rabbits, guinea fowl, (granule are eosinophilic)

Characters

- Cells short lived in circulation, reach affected area to phagocytose foreign bodies
- Neutrophilia: increase in number of neutrophils in the circulation
- **Schilling index**-assess the number of immature neutrophils (band is less/ lacking)
- Shift to left- Immature neutrophils are more in count.

- **Toxic neutrophils (Dohle bodies)**
  - Less chemotactic response
  - Vacuoles of varying size, beginning in Golgi apparatus
  - Granules-Dense and heavy stained seen in systemic diseases, fever and septicaemias

Morphology/ Character

10 – 20 µm in diameter in size.

Blood: Ruminants-30-40%; Monogastric animals- 60-70%

Segmented nucleus (3-5 segments) (PMN) Cytoplasm eosinophilic

Granules in cytoplasm rich in lysosomal enzymes

Rapid amoeboid movement

Aggressive phagocytosis

Granules-two types

1. **Smaller specific (secondary):** Granules contains lysozyme, collagenase, gelatinases, lactoferrin, plasminogen activator, histaminases, ALP, etc., some lipase (lack in macrophages) secrete extra cellularly,
2. **Larger azurophilic (primary)** granules have myeloperoxidase, lysozyme, defensins-bactericidal factors, acid hydrolases, many neutral proteases-non specific cathepsins, elastases, cathepsin G, etc .Highly destructive released within in cells into phagosome.

Origin

- Granulocyte colony stimulatory factor (G-CSF) from different cells induce neutrophil production.

- Myeloid tissue of bone marrow
- Attracted to injured area by chemotaxis (C3,C5)
- No reproduction at inflammatory site

Condition Encountered

- Acute inflammation
- First line of cellular defense
- Pyogenic organisms infected
- Increased in early inflammatory response

Functions

- Phagocytosis
- Highly chemotactic
- Killing and destruction of bacteria and dead cells through liposomes and proteolytic enzymes
- Energy source for other cells (MNC)

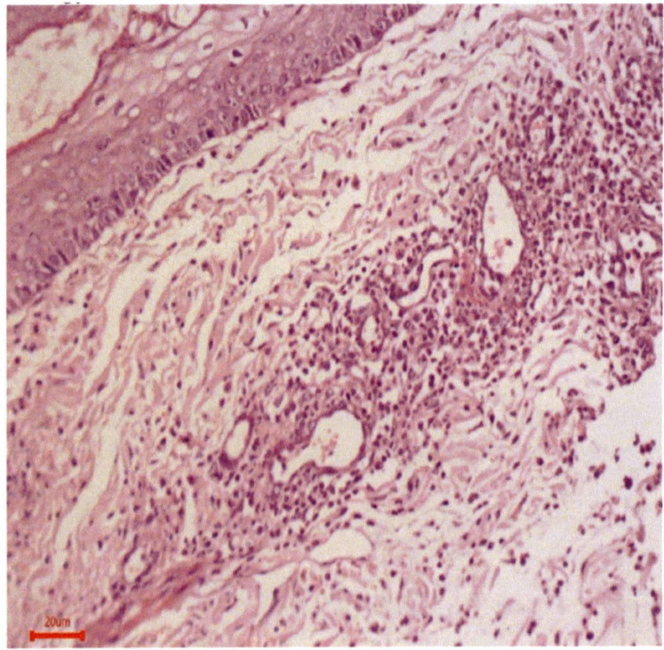

Skin-Dermis-Neutrophilic infiltration

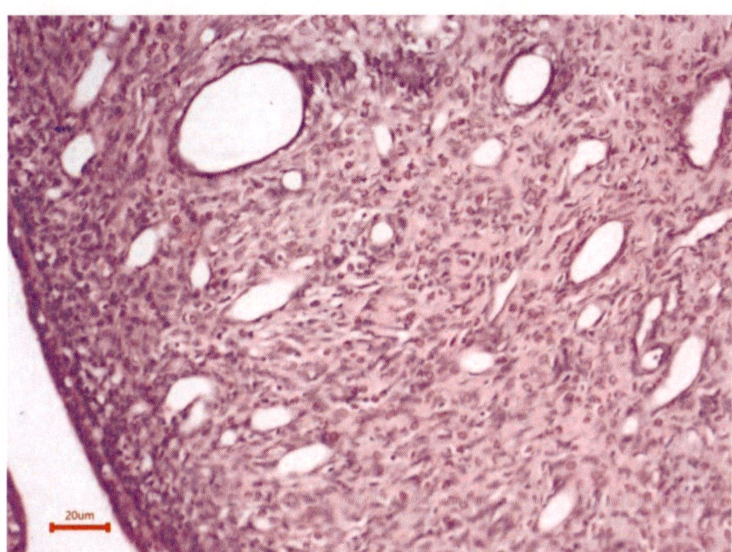

Uterus-Neutrophilic infiltration

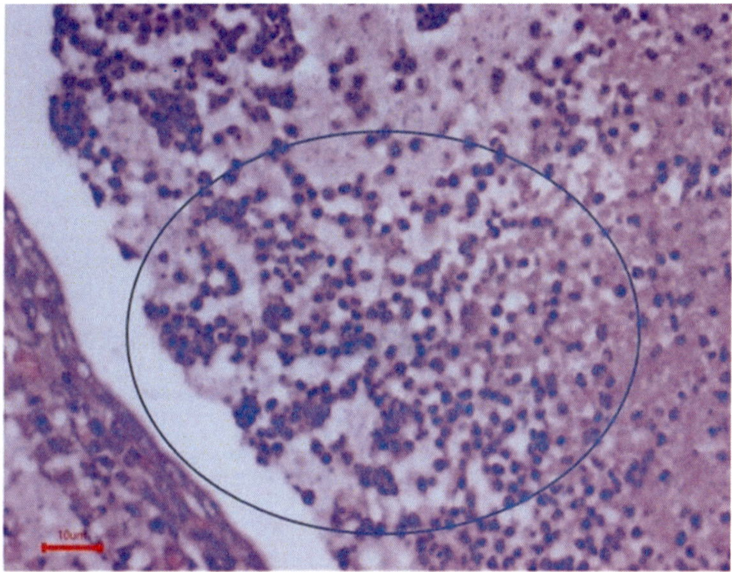

Acute inflammation-Neutrophils (Circle)

Eosinophils

Morphology / Characters

- Domestic animals, circulation present between 1-7%
- 10 – 15 µm in diameter in size
- Nucleus – Bilobed
- Cytoplasmic granules are large and eosinophilic and contain basic protein (toxic to parasite)
- Short lived , found in tissue fluid, skin, intestine, respiratory tract, epithelial linings
- Motile, sluggishly phagocytic, chemotactic (Similar to neutrophils)
- Major Basic Protein (MBP) -Beneficial when toxic to parasites, but can cause tissue damage; lyse membrane epithelial cells
- Chemotaxis- Eotaxin-CCR-3-Surface receptors in eosinophils

Origin

- Myeloid tissue of bone marrow
- No reproduction at site of inflammation

Conditions

- Eosinophilia-Increase in number in circulation
- Appear late in inflammation
- Most prominent in conditions where there is no immune response. e.g., hay fever, asthma in man, parasitic conditions
- Allergy-Immune reaction-IgE antibody
- Parasitic infections especially invasive and migrating phases of parasitic infection and attracts eosinophils

Functions

Eosinophils granules

S.No.	Granules contain	Functions
i	Major Basic Protein (MBP)	Highly charged cationic protein-Toxic to parasites; Lysis of epithelial cells
ii	Eosinophilc cationic proteins (ECP)	Direct toxicity to parasitic cuticle and epithelial cells Degranulation on parasitic cuticle
iii	Eosinophilic peroxidase (EP)	Oxidative stress and tissue damage

- Produce leukotrienes on activation (LTC4) and PAF, that can amplify and sustain inflammatory response
- Chemotactic
- Phagocytic – killing parasite
- Hypersensitivity reactions

Eosinophilic Granulomas of Domestic Animals

Species	Type of Eosinophilic Granuloma
Feline	Eosinophilic plaque, granuloma, and dermatitis
Canine	Eosinophilic granuloma of the oral cavity of Huskies and other dogs
Equine	Equine collagenolytic granuloma, axillary nodular necrosis, and unilateral popular dermatosis
All species	Eosinophilic (TH2) granulomas secondary to parasitic infections

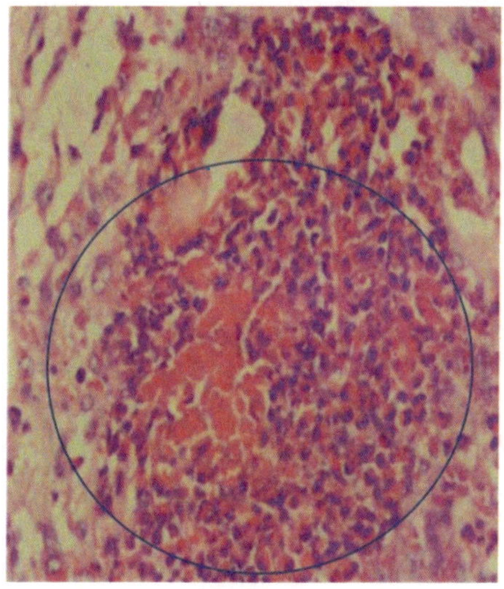

Eosinophils (Circle) infiltrating around lysed collagen

Basophils

Perivascular location -Lung, brain, skin, Intestine (diarrhoea)

Morphology / Character

- Found in blood (0.5 to 1%)
- 10 – 15 μm in diameter in size
- Similar to mast cell, cytoplasmic granules, cell surface (IgE Fc receptors etc) IgE sensitized cells
- Early stage of inflammation
- Exposure to UV irradiation, trauma, heat and cold,
- Degranulation occurs and sustained by C3a and C5a (anaphylotoxins) eosinophil peroxidase
- Differ from mast cells as basophils have multilobed nuclei, dense peripheral chromatin, less numerous large granules, less complex cell surface
- Motile
- Non-phagocytic
- Seen in small numbers in inflammation
- Large lobulated nuclei
- Granules contain heparin and histamine but no acid hydrolases, TNFα, eosinophils/neutrophil/ chemotactic factor (ECF/NCF), neutral proteases
- Involved in Type -I hypersensitivity reaction

Mast Cells

- Widely distributed in connective tissue
- Produces early vascular changes
- Acute inflammation through histamine and arachidonic acid metabolites (LT &PG) Refer to chemical mediators for details
- Mononuclear cell
- Larger in size about 20 μm in diameter in size
- Abundant cytoplasm

- Granules contain heparin, histamine and proteolytic enzymes
- Some animals, rich in serotonin
- Have Fc receptor for IgE antibody (Fc ERC)

Functions

Both basophils and mast cells release heparin / histamine in response to Ag – Ab complexes

The immunoglobulin IgE binds selectively to the surface of mast cells and basophils

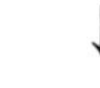

Triggers degranulation

Release of histamine and other mediators, anaphylaxis (C3a and C5a anaphlyotoxins)-Catastrophic

In acute inflammation

- Trauma
- UV light
- Heat
- Cold
- Food
- Insect venom
- Drugs

Lymphocytes

Morphology / Characters

- In circulation -Ruminants: About 60-70%; dogs 30-40%
- 7 – 12 μm in diameter in size
- Nucleus round
- Having compact chromatin within the nucleus
- Cytoplasm invisible or

- Cytoplasm, homogenous, pale blue and may contain a few azurophil granules

Origin

- Two lymphocytic population - T lymphocytes (found in circulation) → Cell mediated immunity
- B lymphocytes transform into plasma cells which are involved in humoral immunity.
- When they come in contact with antigen and produce antibodies – Humoral immunity

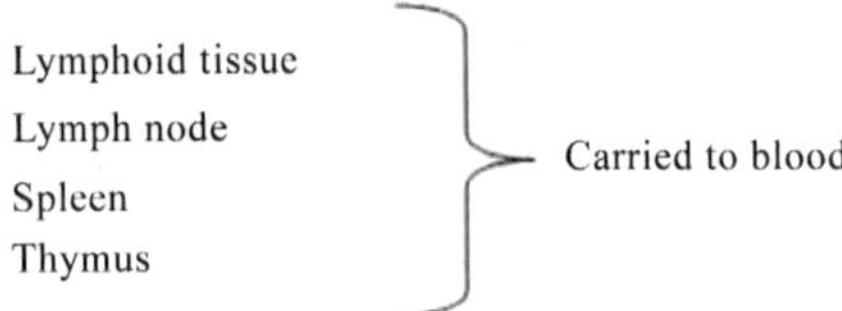

Bursa of Fabricius-Birds-B- lymphocytes

Conditions

- Occurs late in inflammation 48 – 72 hours
- Viral infections particularly in CNS
- Brain and spinal cord → Perivascular cuffing
- **Perivascular cuffing:** Being slightly amoeboid in movement, the lymphocytes just come out of blood vessels and surround the vessels characteristically seen in brain in Rabies and avian encephalomyelitis
- Endocrine secretions from pituitary and adrenal cortex control the number of lymphocytes e.g. glucocorticoids

Functions

- Humoral and cell mediated immunity

Plasma Cells

- **Not found in circulation**
- 12 – 15 μm in size
- Round to oval cells
- Nucleus similar to lymphocytes, eccentric

- Cart - wheel like arrangement of nuclear chromatin
- Cytoplasm abundant
- Slightly amoeboid and phagocytic

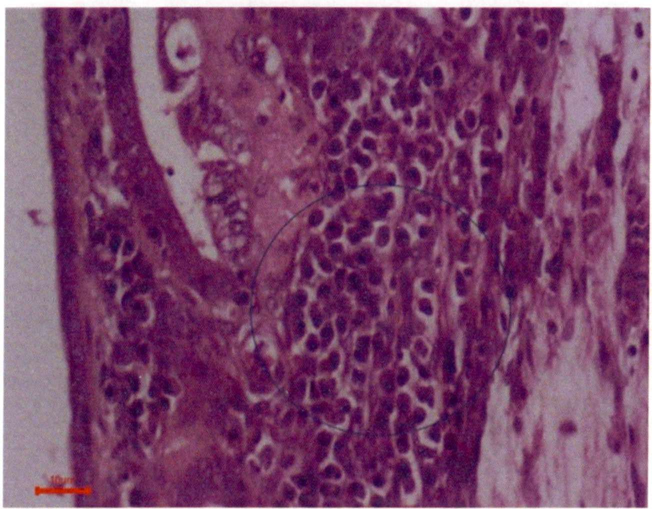

Plasma cells (Circle)

Origin

- From B-lymphocytes
- Function -Antibody production.

Macrophages

Synonyms

- Macrophages of Metchnikoff
- Second line of cellular defense

Morphology/ Character

- 12 – 20 µm diameter in size
- Nucleus round to oval
- 1 – 2 nucleoli
- Macrophages may bunch together to form giant cells
- Amoeboid and phagocytic

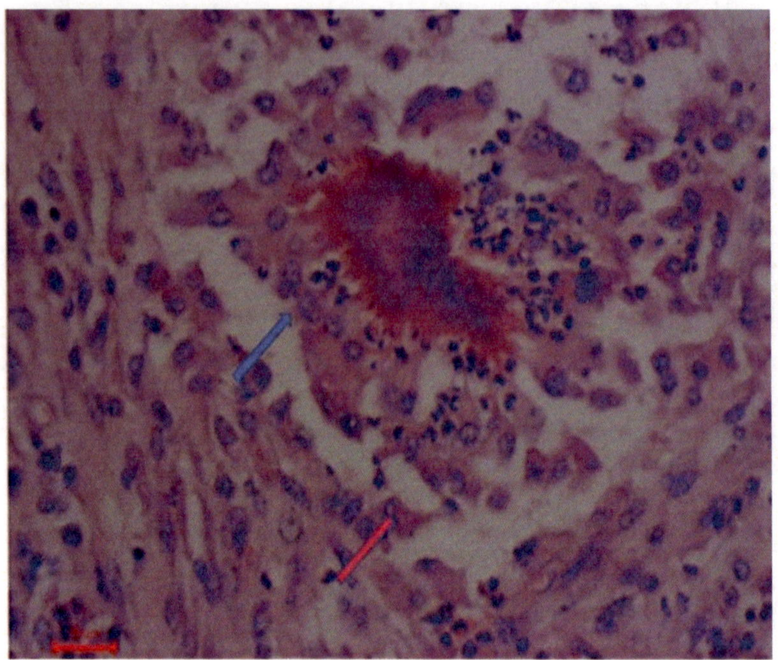

Macrophage (Blue arrow); Epithelioid cell (Red arrow)

Origin

- Macrophages originate from monocytes
- Monocytes emigrate from the blood into the inflammatory lesions and transform into macrophages
- Capable of reproduction at the site of inflammation

Monocytic phagocytic system

- Histiocytes - Connective tissue
- Kupffer cells - Liver
- Microglial cells –Nervous system
- Alveolar macrophages - Lung
- Fixed / free macrophages -Spleen / lymphnode
- Skin -Langerhans's cell
- Bone -Osteoclasts

Macrophages (Macrophage of Metchnikoff) + Monocytes - Mononuclear Phagocytic System

Macrophage – Prima donna of chronic inflammation closely related cells of bone marrow origin

These cells contain

Monocular phagocytic system (MPS)

Macrophages contain/produce

1. Enzymes

   Elastase

   Collagenase

   Plasminogen activator

   Acid hydrolases

   Phosphatases

   Lipases

2. Plasma proteins

   Complement components (C1 to C5, properdin)

   Coagulation factors (factors V, VIII, tissue factor)

3. Reactive metabolites of oxygen
4. Arachidonic acid (AA) metabolites (leukotrienes, prostaglandins)
5. Cytokines, chemokines (IL-1, TNF, IL-8)
6. Growth factors (PDGF, FGF, TGF-beta), and
7. Nitric oxide (NO)

Derived from monocytes (Blood 3-5%)
Monocytes in blood has half-life of one day

↓

Growth differentiation factors, cytokines, adhesion molecules, cell – interaction

↓

Reach tissue (life span several months- Tissue macrophages are widely distributed)

↓

Arrive 48 hours later in inflammation

↓

Extravasation (Similar to neutrophils)

Condition Encountered

- Arrives 48 – 72 hours in inflammation (Second line of cellular defense)
- Late arrival
- Response to immune mediated reaction, endotoxin, fibronectin, chemical mediators.
- Activated T cells secretes gamma interferons which activates macrophages

Functions

- Second line of cellular defense
- Phagocytosis
- Chemotactic
- Produce potent enzymes that degrade connective tissue
- Release substances responsible for fever & leucocytosis (prostaglandins, endogenous pyrogens)
- Release factors in wound healing
- Secrete lysosymes, interferon defense mechanism
- Serves to process antigens in CMI

Modified/transformed macrophages are

1. Epithelioid cells
2. Giant cells (multinucleated cells)

Epithelioid Cells

In H & E-stained section, these cells show pale pink granular cytoplasm with indistinct cell borders, often appearing to merge with one another.

Nucleus of these cells dense than lymphocyte, oval or elongate and may show folding membrane.

Giant Cells

Multinucleated cells formed by fusion of macrophages

Foreign Body Giant Cell

- Fusion of macrophages evoked in response to foreign body
- Contain 50 – 100 nuclei
- Nuclei arranged in periphery of cells (horse-shoe pattern)

  e.g. Langhan's giant cell → TB

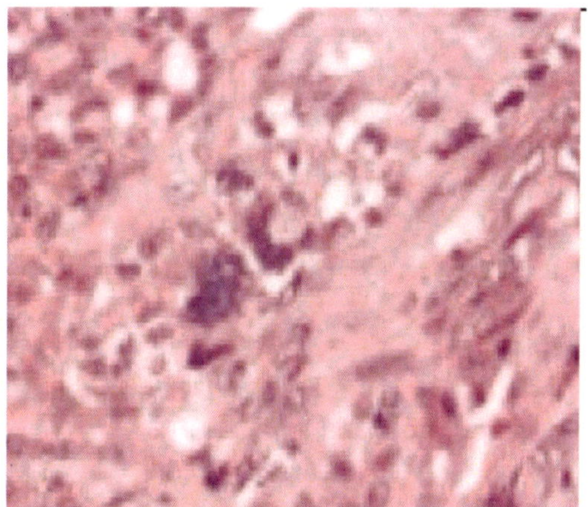

Giant cell-Langhan's type-Horse -shoe arrangement of nuclei-Tuberculosis

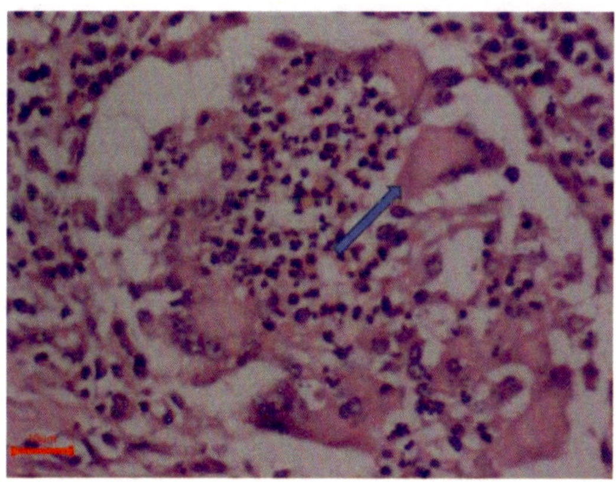

Foreign Body Giant Cell (Blue arrow); Note neutrophils at the centre

Tumor – Giant Cell

Nuclear division without cytoplasmic division. Nuclei may be scattered or found in one or both poles.

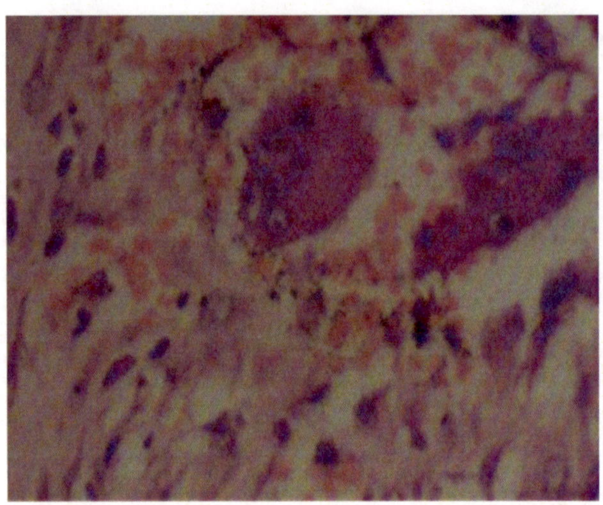

Tumour Giant Cell-Dog-Fibrosarcoma

Reed – Sternberg Cells

Hodgkin's disease (mirror image nuclei – two)

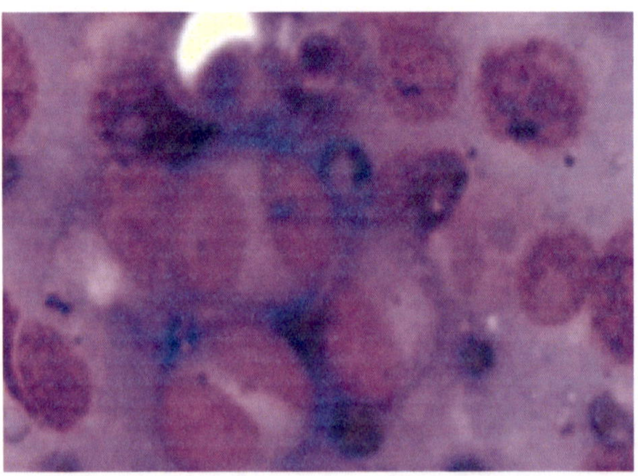

Hodgkin's lymphoma-Reed Sternberg Giant cell-Mirror-image nuclei (Courtesy: Dr. M. Thangapandiyan)

Touton Giant Cell

Ring like arrangement of nuclei e.g. Xanthomas

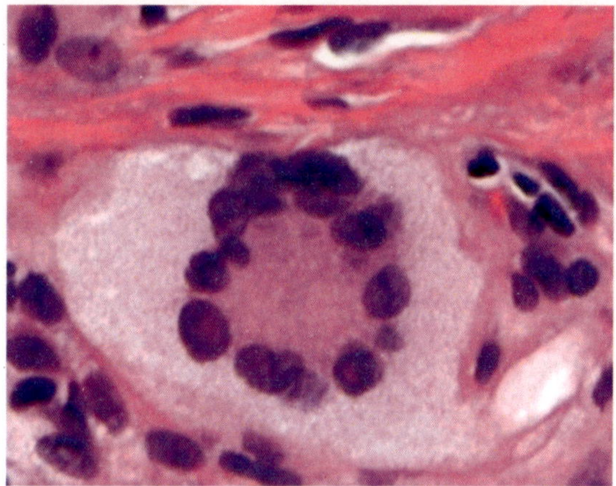

Touton giant cell- Nuclei are arranged in the periphery of the cell- Xanthoma *Courtesy*: Internet -Wikipedia

Systemic Effects of Inflammation

a. Fever
b. Suppression of fever
c. Leukocytic response

Fever

Fever is the main response in acute inflammation.

Definitions

- Abnormal elevation of body temperature due to systemic disturbances
- Fever is a complex systemic response that includes increased body temperature, respiration and heart rate.
- It is a syndrome of elevated body temperature increased due to that effect of potent cytokines released by inflammatory cells.

1. Increase in the body temperature

2. Mechanism

- The endogenous pyrogens of leucocytic origin elevate hypothalamic thermostat.
- Bacterial products, immune complexes, toxins, physical injury, other cytokines

- Macrophage (and other cell) activation
- IL-1 / TNF
- Activate through hypothalamic thermoregulatory centre

3. Effects of Fever

1. Acute phase reactions

a. Fever – increased sleep, decreased appetite
b. Increased acute phase proteins
c. Haemodynamic effects (shock)
d. Neutrophilia

2. Endothelial effects

a. Increased leucocyte adhesion
b. Increased PGI synthesis
c. Increased procoagulant activity
d. Decreased anticoagulant activity
e. Increased IL-1,IL-6, IL-8, PDGF

3. Fibroblast effects

a. Increased proliferation
b. Increased collagen synthesis, increased collagenase
c. Increased protease, increased PGE synthesis

4. Leukocyte effects

a. Increased cytokine secretion (IL-1, IL-6)

The progression of fever depends upon

a. Release of pyrogen from leucocytes
b. Suppression of body heat loss by cutaneous vasoconstriction
c. Increased heat production and shivering

Cause of fever includes

a. Bacteria (endotoxin - lipopolysaccharide of gram negative bacteria (multiple causes)

b. Viruses

c. Protozoa

d. Fungi

e. Rickettsia

f. Hypersensitivity reaction (antigen - antibody complexes) - stimulate pyrogen release

g. Mechanical injury - severe crushing, major surgery

h. Vascular disorders - infarction

i. Neoplasm

Clinical effects in mammals

a. Anorexia

b. Somnolescence

c. Malaise

d. Shivering and search for warmth (chills)

The following changes occur in fever

Metabolic changes: 1. Secretion of acute phase proteins, 2. endocrine changes: Increased level of glucocorticoids, growth hormone and aldosterone and decreased vasopressin and **3. Autonomic changes**: Increased blood pressure, pulse rate and decreased sweating.

The most important thermoregulatory mechanism is a redirection of blood flow to skin to deep capillary bed i.e. intended to decrease heat loss from body surface.

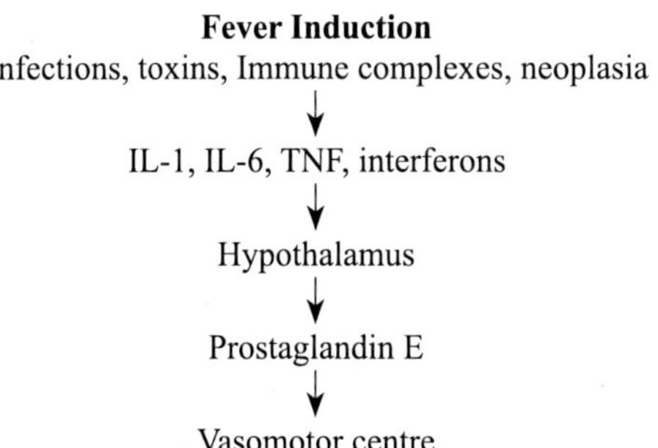

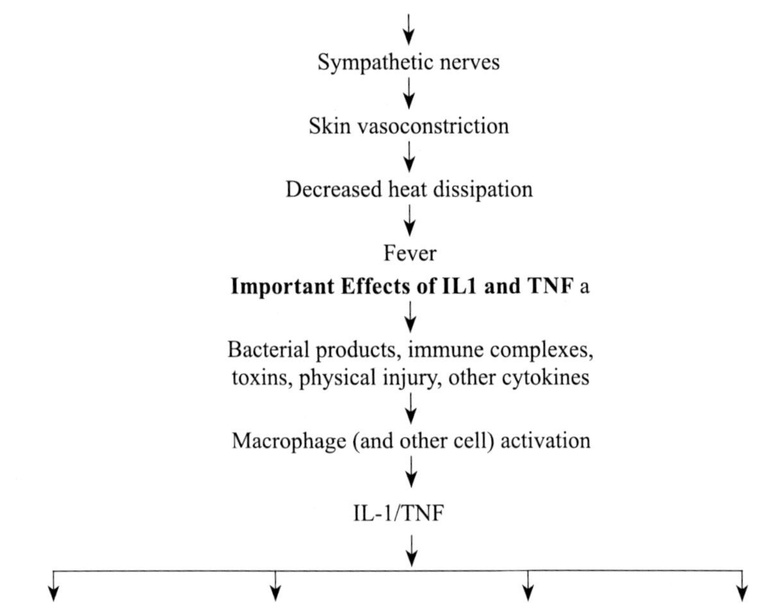

Acute phase reactions	**Endothelial effects**	**Fibroblast effects**	**Leukocyte effects**
Fever	Increased Leukocyte adherence	Increased proliferation	Increased Cytokine Secretion (II-1, IL-6)
Increased sleep Decreased appetite	Increased PGI synthesis	Incrased collagen synthesis Increased collagenase	
Increased acute-phase proteins			
Haemodynamic effects (shock)	Increased procoagulant activity Decreased anticoagulant activity	Increased protease Increased PGE syntheiss	
Neutrophilia	Increased IL-1, IL-6, IL-8, PDGF		

IL 1 – Interleukin 1;TNF-a - Tumour necrosis factor alpha;PDGF – Platelet derived growth factor; PGE – Prostaglandin E;PI – prostatlandin I

12

Healing (Tissue Repair)

Tissue – Proliferating Potential of Cell Types

1. Labile Cells

- Continuously dividing cells
- e.g. epidermis, epithelial cells, bone marrow cells

2. Stable Cells - Quiescent cells

- Undergoes division occasionally
- Liver, kidney pancreas, fibroblasts,
- Endothelial cells

3. Permanent Cells - Non–dividing cells: Neurons, muscle cells (cardiac, skeletal)

According to their proliferative capacity, these cells are regenerated in loss or replaced /substituted by other cell

Wound healing occurs by

i) Regeneration ii) Substitution

Wound healing

Wound healing is not a separate process and occurs along with the inflammatory reaction.

It is a complex but orderly phenomenon involving a number of processes. Namely

1. Acute inflammatory reaction following initial injury
2. Parenchymatous cellular regeneration
3. Migration and production of parenchymatous and connective tissue cell

4. Extracellular matrix, protein synthesis
5. Remodelling of connective tissue

Healing by Primary Union or First Intention

- This type of healing occurs in clean surgical approximated incision i.e. limited bleeding and tissue destruction.

The sequence of events occurring in primary union is given below

0th Hour	Clot filling the incised area
3-24 hour	Neutrophilic infiltration
48 hour	Basal cell proliferation and epithelial closure takes place by 24-48 hours
72 hours	Macrophages replace neutrophils. Granulation tissue begins to appear. Collagen is arranged vertically
120 hours	Incised space is filled with granulation tissue. Neovascularisation is maximal. Collagen fibre begin to appear and epithelial proliferation is maximal

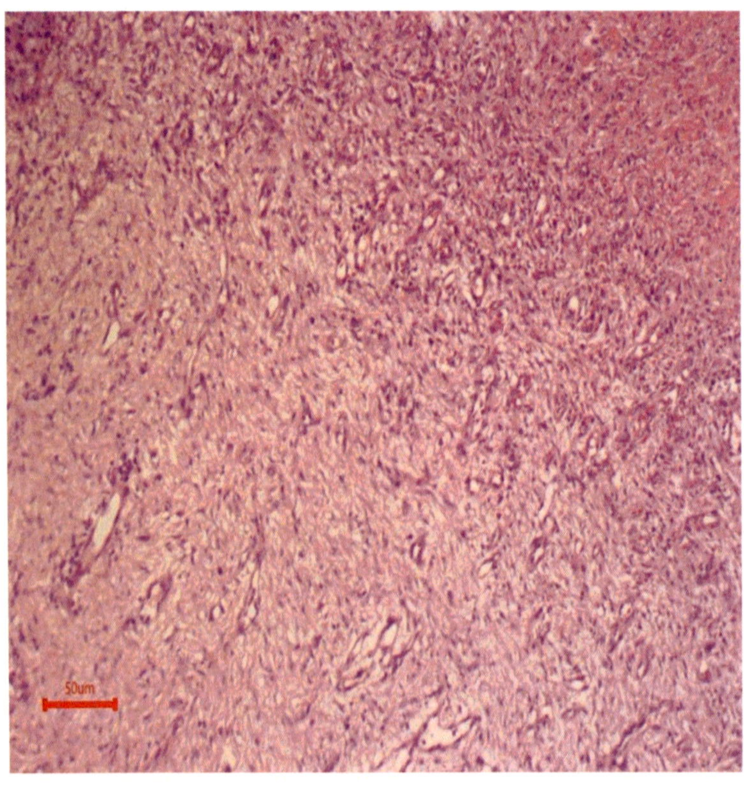

Granulation tissue -Skin

Healing By Second Intention

- The wound involved shows extensive loss of cells and tissue. e.g. infarction, ulceration, abscesses, surface wound with large defects.
- The wound is filled with tissue debris, a few erythrocytes and bacteria.
- Abundant granulation tissue (soft, pink, granular appearance of wound surfaces) grows in from the margin to fill the defect but at the same time the wound contracts i.e., the defect is marked by depression and decrease from its original size.
- Microscopically granulation tissue consists of new capillaries, fibroblasts, collagen and proteoglycan rich ground substance. Initially granulation tissue is soft and spongy due to leaky blood vessels.

Sequential Events in Healing by Second Intention

Injury – open wound – excess loss of tissue – infected – necrosis – inflammation

↓

Blood clot

↓

24 hours – neutrophils infiltrate to destroy irritant

↓

48-72 hours – macrophages and lymphocytes infiltrate

↓

Removal of necrotic and cellular debris by liquefaction by macrophages

↓

120 h-Red granules from underneath (granulation tissue) represent proliferating capillaries.

Fibroblast also proliferate to fill the gap

↓

There is a definite order.

Base - capillaries grow vertically and project towards the surface (Angiogenesis; neovascularization). Fibroblast grows perpendicular to capillary and parallel to surface – pulling pressure of the wound

↓

Surface – fibroblasts are arranged parallel to capillaries exerting tension towards wound surface for easy closure. This arrangement differentiates granulation tissue from fibrosarcoma which lacks orderly arrangement

↓

The surface is closed by the epithelium proliferating from the margin

↓

2nd week proliferation of fibroblast and collagen deposition

↓

2 week- Proliferation of fibroblast with continuous collagen accumulation producing a scar. Type III collagen is deposited early in scar tissue and is replaced by adult type I collagen which accounts for wound strength. Newly formed blood vessels disappear.

8th week- Scar tissue consists of granulation tissue which is devoid of inflammation covering intact epidermis.

The tissue is devoid of sweat gland, sebaceous gland, hair and hair follicles and pigment. So, the scar appears dry and unpigmented white and puckered as it becomes avascular and shrinkage of collagen.

Inflammation and newly formed vessels disappear Type II is early collagen; Type I is adult collagen, accounting for wound strength

3rd month

- Wound strength -70-80% of normal tissue
- Here damaged tissue is replaced by fibrous tissue.
- The process in which are angiogenesis, neovascularization, fibrosis and scar remodeling. These influenced by various factors, growth factors (dealt separately), enzymes and certain nutritional factors.
- Angiogenesis: bFGF and VEGF influences endothelial proliferation of blood vessels , break basement membrane by proteins to reach wound site and vascular tissue formation,
- Fibrosis: proliferation of fibroblast induced by growth factors (PDGF, FGF, TGF-beta) and collagen synthesis
- Remodeling scar: extra cellular matrix (ECM-amorphous collagen, proteoglycan, fibrinonectin) in scar is degraded, modified and remodeled
- Metalloproteinases especially Zn, cleave type I, II and III to fibrillar collagen

Matrix Metalloproteinase Activity, Regulation, and cellular production

Function	Collagenases, gelatinases, stromelysins, matrilysin, enamelysin, metalloelastase, membrane MMPs, inducers of transcription
Cofactors necessary	Zinc [Zn2+]
Regulation	Cellular synthesis, lysosomal degradation and release and tissue inhibitors of metalloproteinases [TIMPs1-4]
Model	Cell type of MMP
MMP 1,2,3,11,14	Fibroblasts
MMP 9,12	Macrophages
MMP 9	Neutrophils
MMP2,3,9	Endothelial cells
MMP 9	Pericytes
MMP 1, 3, 7 ,9 13	Some cancer cells

- And gelatinase type IV collagen
- Remodeling controlled by Tissue Inhibitors Metalloproteinases-TiMPs

Exuberant granulation or proud flesh

- Sometimes the granulation continues to grow with abnormally large amount due to irritant, movement or trauma which prevents healing.
- This condition is called proud flesh or excess granulation tissue.

Keloid

- Keloid is another condition. Reason for its development is not known.
- The connective tissue below the epithelial covering continues to proliferate.
- This condition may recur after the removal.
- This is found in horses and black people having some genetic or familial predisposition.

Systemic and Local Factors Influencing Wound Healing

Systemic Factors

1. Nutritional Factors

a. Vitamins – Vitamin C is required for collagen synthesis which convert proline to hydroxyl proline and lysine to hydroxyl lysine. Vitamin C deficiency will result in little collagen production by fibroblast or of poor quality collagen

b. Proteins deficiency – Starvation- especially methionine and cysteine are required for wound tensile strength affect formation of fibroblast and cathepsins and wound healing

c. Sulphur containing amino acids (methionine and cystine) are important and required for intermediate forms of collagen

d. Zinc – as metalloenzyme, it is essential for remodelling of extracellular matrix (ECM)- Zn deficiency - delayed wound healing. Supplementation Zn will restore the condition

2. Metabolic factors

a. Diabetes mellitus – delays healing

b. Hyperadrenocortism- Glucocorticoids -anti-inflammatory and inhibits collagen synthesis affects wound healing

3. Circulatory stasis or adequacy of blood supply

    a. Inadequate blood supply – delays healing

4. Hormones – concurrent glucocorticoid therapy hinders inflammatory and reparatory process

Local Factors

1. Infection can delay healing
2. Mechanical – Movements directly affect wound healing
3. Foreign bodies impede healing.
4. Size, location and type of wound
5. Cold inhibits wound healing.

Others

1. Old age-Healing is slower than young ones.
2. Chemotherapeutic agents
3. Radiation
4. Immunodeficiency

Collagen biosynthesis

(Most common protein in extracellular matrix-giving frame work)

Cell

↓

Nucleus

↓

DNA

mRNA splicing

↓

RNA

↓

RER Requires Vitamin C

Hydroxylation of proline and lysine

↓

Procollagen (hydroxyproline)

↓

Glycosylation

↓

Golgi apparatus (Procollagen aligned to form triple helix) (procollagen-poly peptide)

Secreted

↓

Extracellular space

↓

Procollagen chipping terminal propeptide

↓

Trophocollagen (Fibre)

Oxidation of lysine and hydroxylysine

↓

Lysyl oxidase

↓

cross linkage result between alpha chain

↓

Stabilizing array i.e. characteristic of collagen

(Cross linkage is the major contributor for tensile strength of collagen)

Cell Cycle and Cyclins

- Proliferation of cells are important in degeneration and repair and also a feature in neoplasia.
- The dividing cells undergo cyclical change i.e cell cycle and it has four phases.

1. Presynthetic growth phase or G1 phase – This is the time gap between end of mitosis and start of DNA synthesis.
2. Synthetic phase or S phase – This is period of DNA synthesis and beginning of mitosis.
3. A premitotic growth phase or G2 phase
4. Mitotic phase or M phase

- A cell takes 24 hours to give rise to another cell.

The time taken by different phases is as follows phases

Time taken	(hours)
G1	11
S	8
G2	4
M	1
	24

- The cell is usually in interphase and G1 is most variable period. G0 state wherein cell proliferation is arrested.
- The cyclins synthesized during specific phase of cell cycle are involved in activating cyclin dependant kinases (CDK).
- Once the job is completed, the cyclins leave their activity. This is the way the cell cycle or proliferation is regulated.
- G1 to S phase is regulated by cyclin D/CDK4, cyclin D/CDK6, cyclin D/CDK2.
- S phase is regulated by cyclin D/CDK2, cyclin A/CDK1.
- G2 to M phase transistion is regulated by cyclin B/CDK1.
- Cyclin D gene sare overexprssed in many cancers so that neoplastic transformation occurs. e.g.hepatic tumour, breast cancer.
- Cell cycle is also regulated by CDK inhibitors. e.g. CDKNIA (p21), p27 and p57. The members acting on cyclin D/CDK4 and cyclin D/CDK6 are p15, CDKN2A (p16), p18 and p19.

Cell cycle checkpoints

- Cell cycle checkpoints are used by the cell to monitor and regulate the progress of the cell cycle.

- Checkpoints prevent cell at specific points, allowing verification of necessary phase processes and repair of DNA damage.
- The cell cannot proceed to the next phase until checkpoint requirements have been met.
- The checkpoints are designed to ensure that damaged or incomplete DNA is not passed on to daughter cells.
- Two main checkpoints are: the G1/S checkpoint and the G2/M checkpoint.
- G1/S transition is a rate-limiting step in the cell cycle and is also known as restriction point.
- An alternative model of the cell cycle response to DNA damage has also been proposed, known as the post replication checkpoint.
- p53 plays an important role in triggering the control mechanisms at both G1/S and G2/M checkpoints.

Growth Factors

- Growth factors (GF) act by autocrine, paracrine, endocrine or signaling pathways.
- GFs play a role in the movement of inflammatory cells, in contractility of cells and differentiation in wound healing.
- These are polypeptides found in the serum and/or elaborated by cells.

Four chemical signaling pathways

These are found in multicellular organisms.

1. Autocrine
2. Paracrine
3. Endocrine
4. Direct contact

1. Autocrine

An autocrine signal (acting on itself) is one that binds to receptors on the surface of the cell that produces it. The chemicals produced by the cell acts on the same cell. i.e. Autocrine signaling acts on the signaling cell. Autocrine glands are the glands that produce hormones that act on their own glandular cells, e.g.

prostaglandins. Epidermal growth factor (EGF) and its receptor (EGFR) in epithelial cells. CD4+ T cells use autocrine signaling through interleukin (IL)-2 to control their proliferation and apoptosis.

2. Paracrine

The chemicals produced by the cell acts on the neighbouring cells. i.e. Paracrine signaling acts on nearby cells. Paracrine glands are those whose hormones are released into the extracellular matrix and reach the adjacent cells via diffusion, e.g., islets of Langerhans – somatostatin, ovaries, testes

3. Endocrine

Endocrine signaling uses the circulatory system to transport ligands. i.e. The chemicals, hormones, produced by the cell through circulation reaches target cells and act on them (distant cells). E.g. Pituirary, thyroid, pancreas, goads

4. Direct contact

Signaling via gap junctions involves signaling molecules moving directly between adjacent cells. Responses that last only a short amount of time.

The main growth factors are

1. **Epidermal Growth Factor (EGF):** It is a polypeptide of 6-kDa, a progression factor which acts by combining with EGF receptors in the cell membrane.

   Transforming growth factor-alpha (TGF-α) is homologous to this factor. Both are mitogenic for epithelial cells and fibroblasts.

2. **Platelet Derived Growth Factor (PDGF):** It is stored in platelets and of 30-kDa size.

   PDGF may be released upon activation of platelets, macrophages, endothelium and tumour cells.

   It is a complement factor and requires a progression factor for its activation.

   PDGF is responsible for migration and proliferation of fibroblasts, macrophages and smooth muscle cells.

3. **Fibroblast Growth Factor (FGF):** It includes acidic and basic FGFs.

   These are involved in angiogenesis, cell migration and proliferation of endothelial cells.

Besides, they are involved in wound repair, development and haematopoesis.

Basic FGFs are found in many organs and released by activated macrophages. Acidic FGF is usually found in neural tissue.

4. **Transforming Growth Factor-beta (TGF-β):** It is derived from platelets, endothelium, T cells and macrophages.

   It induces fibrosis by stimulating fibroblast chemotaxis, collagen and fibronectin synthesis and inhibition of collagen degradation.

   It is also inhibitory to most epithelial cells' growth.

5. **Vascular Endothelial Growth Factor (VEGF):** It promotes formation of blood vessels (Angiogenesis), also plays a role in angiogenesis of chronic inflammation and healing of wounds. Specifically, lymphatic endothelial cell proliferation is induced by VEGF.

6. **Tumour necrosis factor-alpha (TNF-α) and Interleukin-1 (IL-1):** These cytokines play a role in fibroplasia by attracting fibroblasts and increasing collagen synthesis. TNF-α is also angiogenic in nature.

13

Immunodficiency Diseases-Syndromes

Definition

IDD (immunodeficiency diseases) occur when there is a failure of the immune system to protect the host from infectious organisms or the development of cancer.

IDD are disorders of immune system that result in immunological deficiency. Immunodeficiency could be from defects in

i. B and T- lymphocytes

ii. Granulocytes

iii. Complement

IDD may be caused by

1. Primary IDD-Hereditary-Genetic- may be inherited or congenital-Defect in development of immune system
2. Secondary IDD-Acquired-Due to infection, aging, malnutrition, immunosuppression, autoimmunity, irradiation and chemotherapy

Hence, immunodeficiency may result in different disease conditions as per the type of defect noticed in the animal.

I. Primary IDD

May be inherited or congenital affecting

1. Specific immunity i.e. Humoral (HI) and cell-mediated immunity (CMI) and involve B- or T-lymphocytes or both or
2. Non-specific immunity i.e., components of innate immune responses like complement, phagocytosis, NK cells etc.

Primary IDD

1. Inherited Defects in Phagocytosis

a. Chediak-Higashi syndrome
b. Pelger-Huet anomaly
c. Canine leukocyte adherence deficiency (CLAD)
d. Bovine leukocyte adherence deficiency (BLAD)

a. Chediak-Higashi syndrome: The disease affects cattle, rats and human beings increasing susceptibility to infection due to abnormally large granules (fusion of lysosomes) in neutrophils, monocytes and eosinophils. The leukocyte granules become fragile and cause tissue damage by rupture. Affected leukocytes are defective in chemotaxis, motility and reduced intracellular killing. The CH syndrome by affecting NK cell development may increase susceptibility to tumours and some viruses.

b. Pelger-Huet anomaly: Inherited defect in neutrophil nuclear segment formation looking like immature cell with rounded nucleus encountered in cattle, dogs, cats and rabbits.

c. Canine LAD: There is an absence of integrins required for adhesion of neutrophils to blood vessel wall resulting in failure of emigration of cells in inflammation. Bacteria are free to spread with recurrent infections are seen.

d. Bovine LAD: Here inherited integrin deficiency occurs in calves with early mortality due to recurrent bacterial infection.

2. Inherited Defects in the Immune System

Genetically determined stem-cell lesion affecting B- and T-lymphocyte production affecting humoral immunity (HI) and cell-mediated immunity (CMI) since thymic and bursal or its equivalent organs do not develop. If defect occurs in T-lymphocyte production antibody production may be normal and CMI is affected. If B-cell production is affected HI is affected.

Severe Combined Immunodeficiency Disease

The SCID is affecting both T and B lymphocytes so HI and CMI are affected. It may be due to autosomal recessive, X-linked or sporadic inherited, encountered in human beings, mice (CB-17 strain, autosomal recessive), dogs (X-linked), cattle (Calf, IgG2 deficiency and hereditary parakeratosis) and horses (Autosomal recessive, Arabian horses, agammaglobulinaemia). There is profound lymphoid hypoplasia of primary (thymus) and secondary lymphoid tissue (Spleen, lymph nodes). It is a family of genetic defects affecting common lymphoid stem cells. Affected animals lack IgG and IgA, and suffer from various bacterial pathogens and die early.

II. Secondary Immunodeficiencies

Various pathogens, toxins, malnutrition and stress may affect immune system with immune deficiencies.

i. **Bacterial infection:** In T-lymphocyte deficiency bacterial sepsis occurs. In B-lymphocyte deficiency, infection is due to Streptococcus and *Staphylococcus* spp. While granulocyte defect may result in *Staphylococcus* spp. and *Pseudomonas* and pyogenic infections in complement defect. *Pasteurella haemolytica* and *Actinobucilli* arc also involved in immunosuppression.

ii. **Viral infections:** In T-lymphocyte deficiency cytomegalovirus, chronic infections with respiratory and intestinal viruses are seen while in B-lymphocyte deficiency enteroviral encephalitis is encountered. IBDV (Infectious bursal disease virus) destroys primary lymphoid organ bursa of Fabricius with failure to produce antibodies. Herpesvirus-1 type in equines (foals) and bovine causes T-cell lymphopaenia and depressed CMI. Retrovirus infection in cats induces lymphoid tumours than other domestic animals. Feline leukemia virus (FeLV) causes lymphocyte destruction and their function and immune complexes causing glomerulonephritis. FeLV-AIDS virus impairs function of T-helper cells. FIV (Feline immunodeficiency virus) occurring in older male cats may cause lymphomas, squamous cell carcinomas and myeloproliferative diseases, immunodeficiency and neurological disease. Retrovirus infections in cattle and dogs also cause immunodeficiency.

iii. **Fungal and parasitic infections:** Candididasis and *Pneumocystis* carinii infections are found in TC-cell deficiency and intestinal giardiasis and aspergillosis in B-cell defect and candidiasis, nocardiasis and aspergillosis may occur in granulocytic deficiency. Immunosuppression may also occur in toxoplasmosis, trypanosomiasis, trichinellosis and demodecosis.

iv. **Toxins:** Environmental toxic pollutants like dieldrin, methyl mercury, iodine, lead, DDT etc., mycotoxins (Aflatoxin, T-2 toxins) are immunosuppressive.

v. **Malnutrition:** Severe nutritional deficiencies also affect immune function.

S. No.	Deficient nutrient	Affect
1.	Vitamin A, B12, folic acid	IgG production through T-cell, CMI
2.	Vitamin D	Macrophage development
3.	Mg	B-cell
4.	Zn, Cr, Se	Immune function
5.	Cu	Neutrophil numbers and function

vi. **Exercise:** Moderate regular exercise boosts immune function while intensive strenuous exercise results in immunodeficiency.

vii. **Trauma:** Severe trauma and burn injuries corticosteroids, prostaglandins from injured tissues and active peptides in serum cause immunosuppression.

viii. **Age:** T-cells (CD4+) may be reduced as age advances but not B-cells. However, aged macrophages show reduces cytokine production. These will cause immunodeficiency.

III. Other conditions

Aggressive disease with opportunistic pathogens, failure to clear infections and adverse reactions to attenuated vaccines in T-cell defect, chronic recurrent GIT infections, sepsis and meningitis in B-cell deficiency and neutrophilia can occur.

14

Hypersensitivity

Definition

Hypersensitivity is an altered reaction to a specific antigen that results in pathologic reactions upon the exposure of a sensitized host to that of specific antigen.

Explanation

Hypersensitivity reactions are inappropriate or misdirected responses to a specific antigen that result in harmful reactions upon exposure of a sensitized host to that specific antigen.

Affected animals require a sensitization phase in which the animal must have had either a previous exposure or a prolonged exposure to the antigen so that it can develop an immune response to the inciting antigen.

The harmful effects resulting from hypersensitivity reactions occur in the effector phase and are most commonly manifested through inflammation or cell lysis.

Classification

Four types are described

1. Type I hypersensitivity
2. Type II hypersensitivity
3. Type III hypersensitivity
4. Type IV hypersensitivity

Based on immunologic mechanisms

That mediates the disease

1. Type I, II and III are mediated by antibody
2. Type IV is mediated by macrophages and T-lymphocytes

1. Type I Hypersensitivity [Immediate hypersensitivity, anaphylactic, allergic (Atopic forms) type].

Type I hypersensitivity is most often the result of an immunoglobulin (Ig): E response directed against environmental or exogenous antigens called allergens, causing the release of vasoactive mediators from IgE-sensitized mast cells and an acute inflammatory response.

On first exposure to an allergen there is an induction of CD4+ T-cells of Th2: type which secrete cytokines IL-4 and IL-5 that may cause IgE production by B-cells, bind to Fc receptors on mast cells and basophils and re-exposure of host to the same antigen results in cross-linking of antigen with cell-bound IgE on mast cell surface, release primary and secondary mediators from mast cells with initial response and result in mast cells growth and production of IL-3 & 5 by mast cells which in turn recruit and activate eosinophil which release granules causing late-phase reaction. However, IgE antibody is protective in parasitic infections.

There are two forms

i. **Systemic** e.g. Anaphylaxis as in bee sting or drugs (penicillin)-Within a few minutes of exposure to sensitized host, pruritus, urticarial, skin erythema develop and the profound respiratory difficulty (bronchoconstriction and aggravated by hypersecretion of mucus). Entire GI musculature is affected resulting in vomiting, abdominal cramps and diarrhoea.

ii. **Localized** as per route of exposure – Skin contact (Allergic dermatitis; urticarial); GI tract (Ingestion; diarrhoea); Lung (Inhalation; bronchoconstriction)

2. Type II Hypersensitivity (Antibody dependent, cytotoxic hypersensitivity- ACCH)

This type most often occurs when IgG or IgM is directed against either an altered self-protein or a foreign antigen bound to a tissue or cell called hapten causing

i. Destruction of the tissue or cell by antibody-dependent cellular cytotoxicity or complement-mediated lysis (direct lysis) or

ii. Altered cellular function without evidence of tissue or cell damage- cells coated with antibody and C3b complement (Opsonized enabling phagocytosis)

The antigen is an allergen mediating through IgG and IgM with cell- or matrix associated antigens with cell surface receptors. e.g. Autoimmune haemoytic anaemia, neonatal isoerythrolysis (rare in domestic animals, important in foals)-mother is allogeneic erythrocytes, antibody in colostrum), transfusion reactions (incompatible donor), drug reactions, pemphigus. The production of IgG and IgM binds to antigens on target cell or tissue with phagocytosis or lysis of them by activated complement or Fc receptors or recruitment of leukocytes.

3. Type III Hypersensitivity(Immune complex hypersensitivity)

This type of hypersensitivity is caused by the formation of insoluble antibody-antigen complexes called immune complexes resulting in activation of the complement system (c3a & C5a-anaphylotoxins) and the development of an inflammatory reaction at the sites of immune complex deposition.

The two forms are

i. Generalized e.g. Rheumatoid arthritis, systemic lupus erythematosus

ii. Localized e.g. Cutaneous Arthus reaction (in dogs blue-eye uveitis)

The IgG and IgM mediated reaction against soluble antigen (Bacterial, viral) as in systemic lupus erythematosus, some glomerulonephritis, serum sickness, Arthus reaction. Antigen-antibody complex deposition results in complement activation, recruitment of leukocytes by complement products and Fc receptors and release of enzymes and other toxic molecules. There will be necrotizing vasculitis (Fibrinoid necrosis) and inflammation.

4. Type IV Hypersensitivity(Cell-mediated hypersensitivity, delayed-type hypersensitivity -DTH)

This type is result of activation of sensitized T-lymphocytes to specific antigen.

The resulting immune response is either mediated by

i. Direct cytotoxicity by lymphocytes or by the

ii. Delayed type: Release of cytokines that act primarily through macrophages to produce chronic inflammation.

In this T-lymphocyte mediated immunological reaction directed against. Soluble antigen (Bacterial, viral), contact antigens, cell-associated antigen, there will be contact dermatitis, transplant rejection, tuberculosis and chronic allergic diseases. There is T-lymphocyte activation with release of cytokines and macrophage activation and T-lymphocyte mediated cytotoxicity. We will encounter perivascular cellular infiltrates, edema, cell destruction and granuloma formation.

This type of hypersensitivity is basis for Tuberculin testing in cattle for bovine tuberculosis, Allergic contact hypersensitivity, and Granulomatous inflammatory response.

Delayed-Type Hypersensitivity

Tuberculin reaction is classical example of DTH. DTH is also a major mechanism of defense in intracellular pathogens (*Mycobacterium tuberculosis*). The tuberculin reaction is induced in animals already sensitized to the tubercle bacillus by a prior injection, or infection. After 8 to 12 h of i/d injection of tuberculin (a protein-lipopolysaccharide extract of the tubercle bacillus), a local erythema and hardening (induration) occurs. It reaches a peak of 1-2 cm diameter in 24 to 72 h (hence, delayed) and then slowly subsides. Microscopically, DTH reaction is seen as perivascular accumulation of CD4+ helper T-cells and a few macrophages. Local secretion of cytokines by these mononuclear cells leads to an increase in vascular permeability and leakage of plasma proteins, giving rise to edema and fibrin deposits (cause for induration.

Cytokines in DTH

Cytokines	Actions
IL (Interleukin)-12	Important cytokine of DTH produced by macrophages on their first contact with TB bacillus differentiates Th1 cells. IL-12 produces below mentioned cytokines.
Gamma interferon (IFN-gamma)	Most important; variety of effects; Macrophages-Increased phagocytic activity; Fibrosis Powerful activator of macrophages and their IL-12 secretion and several polypeptide growth factors (PDGF, TGF-α) Activated macrophages express more class II molecules on the surface Growth factors induce fibroblast proliferation and collagen production; Hence fibrosis occurs in sustained macrophage activation.
IL-2	Induce proliferation of T-cells accumulating at DTH site. Majority bystander cells, 10% Ag specific CD4+
Tumour necrosis factor (TNF) and lymphotoxin (TNF-β)	Effect on endothelial cell: 1. Local vasodilatation (increased blood flow) through nitric oxide, prostacyclin 2. MNC attachment through E-Selectin 3. Cytokines induce endothelial cells to secrete chemotactic factors (IL-8) All these enable lymphocyte and monocyte to emigrate to the site of DTH.

15

Autoimmune Diseases

Definition

The animal reacts to its own tissue (endogenous antigen) to incite production of antibodies or sensitized lymphocytes. There is breakage of tolerance to the self-proteins.

- Autoimmune diseases are prevented by elimination of sensitized T and B lymphocytes by the process of apoptosis in the thymus and bone marrow during development **(Central tolerance; clonal deletion**), in the peripheral tissues (Peripheral tolerance) and clonal anergy **(Clonal avoidance)** by defective presentation of cells.
- The tolerance of CD4+ TH cells is critical in preventing autoimmunity.
- Two major autoimmune diseases are thyroiditis and haemolytic anemia. Other conditions are rare in animals

1. Autoimmune Thyroiditis

Causes

- Genetic predisposition (Doberman dogs)
- Autoantibodies
- Lymphocyte mediated mechanisms

Pathogenesis

- Exact mechanism is not known. There is involvement of T lymphocytes.
- Microscopically, thyroid shows interstitial lymphoplasmacytic infiltration with germinal centres. The thyroid follicular epithelial cells are destroyed by T cells in dogs, causing hypothyroidism.

Signs

- Obesity, lethargy, alopecia, hyperlipidosis and pyoderma in dogs.

2. Autoimmune Haemolytic Anaemia

- The disease is characterized by severe haemolytic anaemia and thrombocytopenia, regenerative anaemia with high reticulocyte counts.
- Erythrocytosis occurs following antigen-antibody attachment to the surface membrane of erythtocytes or by removal of such cells by the splenic macrophages.
- There will be low haemoglobin with spherocytosis and direct Coombs test (antiglobulin) is positive.

3. Cryopathic autoimmune haemolytic anaemia (Cold haemagglutinin disease in dogs and horses)

- The dog is anaemic.
- Anaemia is observed only when the animal is having IgM auto-antibodies or exposed to cold.
- Grossly, lesion is seen in the nose, ears and extremities in dogs.
- Microscopically, capillary stasis, agglutination and lysis of erythrocytes are seen.

4. Myasthenia Gravis

- The autoantibodies bind to acetylcholine receptors at motor endplates resulting in progressive muscular weakness and low exercise tolerance.
- Lymphocytic infiltration in synaptic clefts occurs at a later stage interfering with release of acetylcholine and diminishing the total area of postsynaptic contents.
- Congenital disease occurs in Jack Russell and Smooth Fox Terrier dogs.

5. Pemphigus

- It is characterized by bullae formation in the skin and mucous membrane of dogs and humans.
- Oral mucosa is affected in dogs with loss of epithelial cell coherence and acantholysis.
- Autoantibodies are produced against epithelial cell glycopoteins.

- The variant of pemphigus is known as *Pemphigus foliaceus* in which painful skin disease develops in the face and ears.
- The bullae form under the stratum corneum progressing to scabs and alopecia.
- Footpad lesions are common e.g. Bearded collies.
- In autoimmune pemphigoid, antiglycocalyx antibodies are produced against keratinocytes which affect basement membrane of epithelium

6. Idiopathic Polyradiculoneuritis

- It is a group of diseases of inflammation of peripheral nerves, nerve roots and ganglia, characterized by mononuclear cell infiltration, axonal degeneration and axonal reactions in lower motor nerves

7. Idiopathic Polyneuritis in Dogs (Coonhound Paralysis)

- There is ascending symmetrical paralysis beginning 7-14 days after scratches or bites of raccoons, progressed to tetraparesis.
- The animals are alert and show initial signs of weakness to flaccid symmetric quadriplegia and may be segmental demyelination with perivenular lymphoid infiltration in the ventral nerve roots of spinal cord and some peripheral nerves.

8. Neuritis of the cauda equina

- Neuritis of the cauda equine (**Guillain-Barre syndrome-idiopathic polyneuritis, a postinfectious paralytic disease that typically follows Influenza infection**) in which segmental demyelimation is seen in spinal nerve roots of horses.
- Disintegration of myelin and infiltration of mononuclear phagocytes and macrophages into the sacral intradural rootlets, resulting in paralysis of tail and urinary and intestinal sphincters.

9. Systemic Autoimmune Diseases

Canine Lupus Erythematosus

- A rare disease in which progressive haemolytic anaemia, thrombocytopenic purpura, proteinuria and polyarthritis are seen.
- Renal failure causes death due to glomerulonephritis and plasma cell infiltrations.

- Thymus shows medullary lymphoid follicular development.
- Lymphocytic infiltration is seen around the dermal blood vessels of dogs.
- The anaemia is acute with severe haemolysis and positive antiglobulin (Coombs) test.
- Platelet destruction (autoantibodies to platelets) leading to thromnocytopenia purpura is manifested as haematuria, epistaxis, petechiae and ecchymoses in the skin and mucous membrane.

References

Kumar, V., Abbas, A. K. and Aster, J.C. (2015). Robbins and Cotran Pathologic Basis of Disease. 9th Edition, Elsevier, Philadelphia

Sastry, G. A and Rama Rao, P (2020) Veterinary Pathology, 7th Edition, CBS Publishers and Distributors Pvt Ltd., New Delhi.

Vegad, J. L. (2016). A Textbook of Veterinary General Pathology, 2nd Edition, CBS Publishers and Distributors Pvt Ltd., New Delhi.

Zachary, J. F (2022). Pathologic Basis of Veterinary disease. 7th Edition, Elsevier, Missouri.

Index